Handbook of
Cardiac Electrophysiology

A Practical Guide to Invasive EP Studies and
Catheter Ablation

ReMEDICAPUBLISHING

While every effort is made by the publishers and authors to see that no inaccurate or misleading data, opinions or statements appear in this book, they wish to make it clear that the material contained in the publication represents a summary of the independent evaluations and opinions of the authors and contributors. As a consequence, the authors, publishers and any sponsoring company accept no responsibility for the consequences of any such inaccurate or misleading data or statements. Neither do they endorse the content of the publication or the use of any drug or device in a way that lies outside its current licensed application in any territory.

Published by ReMEDICA Publishing Limited
32–38 Osnaburgh Street, London, NW1 3ND, UK

Tel: +44 20 7388 7677
Fax: +44 20 7388 7457
Email: books@remedica.com
www.remedica.com

Publisher: Andrew Ward
In-house editors: Zoe Healey and Helen James
Design: ReGRAPHICA, London, UK
Printed in India by Ajanta Offset, New Delhi

© 2002 ReMEDICA Publishing Limited
Publication date February 2002

ISBN 1 901346 37 4
British Library Cataloguing-in Publication Data
A catalogue record for this book is available from the British Library

Handbook of Cardiac Electrophysiology

A Practical Guide to Invasive EP Studies and Catheter Ablation

Francis D Murgatroyd MA, MRCP
Consultant Cardiologist, Cardiac Electrophysiology Unit
Papworth Hospital, Cambridge, UK

Andrew D Krahn MD, FRCPC, FACC
Assistant Professor, Division of Cardiology
University of Western Ontario
London, Ontario, Canada

George J Klein MD, FRCPC, FACC
Professor and Head, Division of Cardiology

Raymond K Yee MD, FRCPC, FACC
Professor, Division of Cardiology

Allan C Skanes MD, FRCPC
Assistant Professor, Division of Cardiology

University of Western Ontario
London, Ontario, Canada

Foreword by: **William G Stevenson** MD, FACC
Brigham and Women's Hospital
Boston, MA, USA

ReMEDICAPUBLISHING

CONTENTS

Preface

Acknowledgements

Foreword

Abbreviations and Conventions used in this Book

To the outsider, clinical electrophysiology (EP) appears an arcane subspecialty. Other cardiological disciplines, such as coronary intervention and non-invasive imaging, present similar technical challenges, but at least their visual nature allows the newcomer to grasp the essence of what is 'going on'. In the EP laboratory, the newcomer is confronted with an array of electrical equipment, including imaging, stimulating and recording devices and all eyes are on a monitor displaying a multichannel set of high frequency signals. Understanding these signals as they fly past can seem a daunting challenge.

However, those that learn to master this challenge find that EP is a richly rewarding specialty. It is one of the most logical and coherent branches of medicine, and it appeals to the puzzle-solver in us. It is a hands-on discipline that demands technical dexterity, a three-dimensional mind and the ability to apply logic to the analysis of complex data — and all this *in real time*. Catheter ablation also offers the only truly curative therapy in adult cardiology.

The *Handbook of Cardiac Electrophysiology* is aimed at the cardiology or EP fellow starting in the laboratory, and also at the technicians, engineers and nurses working in EP. Additionally, it will provide a useful reference for more experienced practitioners.

In writing the *Handbook*, we have concentrated on 'classical' EP. The reader is taken systematically through the stages of an EP procedure, from equipment and patient preparation, to the basic study, evaluation of the arrhythmic substrate, arrhythmia induction, techniques for differential diagnosis, and finally the principles of catheter mapping and ablation. We have taken a highly visual approach: all the phenomena described are illustrated with both original color figures and corresponding annotated multichannel tracings recorded on modern equipment. For ease of reading we have wherever possible kept these on the same or facing pages.

This book does not attempt to cover the whole of arrhythmology: discussions of cellular mechanisms; non-invasive diagnosis; and drug and device therapy have been deliberately omitted (these are well covered in other texts, which we have cited below). In addition, we strongly recommend regular perusal of the journals to keep up with the latest advances.

We hope the *Handbook* will provide a useful grounding and reference for those working in an EP laboratory. Each chapter of the *Handbook* ends with suggestions for further reading: research papers, review articles and sections from other EP textbooks. Of the latter, we find Prystowsky and Klein [1] to be the most readable general textbook of clinical arrhythmology; Josephson [2] is an in-depth and detailed single-author account of clinical EP; and for a comprehensive multi-author reference, especially relating to basic science, the 'bible' remains Zipes & Jalifé [3].

To learn the puzzle-solving skills that are so much a part of the appeal of EP, there is no substitute for the close study of individual cases. We strongly recommend trainees to get into the habit of reviewing their EP studies in detail, the same day (some of us learned this the hard way), and to seek an explanation for every phenomenon seen. Even the most 'routine' cases usually contain a point of interest. For practice, an excellent collection of unknown intracardiac tracings is to be found in Klein and Prystowsky [4], and stimulating sessions and courses are put on at most of the large scientific meetings.

ACKNOWLEDGEMENTS

This book crystallizes concepts that we have learned over the years from many people, and we thank those who have inspired, encouraged and taught us. We would particularly like to thank John Camm, Ted Cuddy, John Rabson, Edward Rowland, David Ward and Raymond Yee. Most of all, we are indebted to George Klein for instilling in us his passion for EP, and for his patient support during this book's long gestation. We would like to thank the staff of ReMEDICA, in particular Zoe Healey and Helen James, for their patience, flexibility and many skills in supporting this complex project. Finally, we would like to thank Susan and Dee for putting up with the many absences and phone calls that made this transatlantic project possible.

Francis Murgatroyd
Andrew Krahn

1. Prystowsky EN, Klein GJ. In J Dereck, ed. Cardiac arrhythmia: An integrated approach for the clinician. New York: McGraw-Hill, 1994.
2. Josephson ME. Clinical cardiac electrophysiology. Pennsylvania: Lea & Febiger, 1993.
3. Zipes DP, Jalife J. Cardiac electrophysiology from cell to bedside. Philadelphia: WB Saunders, 2000.
4. Klein GJ, Prystowsky EN. Clinical electrophysiology review. New York: McGraw-Hill, 1997.

Cardiac electrophysiology is one of the most interesting, challenging and rewarding pursuits in clinical medicine. The clinical electrophysiology study pioneered by Hein JJ Wellens, Philip Coumel and others has been the key to understanding a wide variety of supraventricular and ventricular arrhythmias in humans. It requires: planning; appropriate responses to expected and unexpected findings; and the ability to synthesize a complex set of findings to arrive at the diagnosis. With the success of catheter ablation, the procedure has evolved from solely a diagnostic procedure to a diagnostic and therapeutic procedure. The fundamentals of interpretation of the electrocardiogram and intracardiac recordings have never been more important. Making a precise and correct diagnosis is the key to a successful outcome, particularly when multiple arrhythmia mechanisms are possible.

This text will provide the reader with an excellent grounding in the fundamentals of conducting and interpreting cardiac electrophysiologic studies. The basics of electrogram recording and filtering, and programmed stimulation protocols are concisely reviewed. A wealth of clear, well-labeled tracings are presented with concise clear descriptions. Illustrations of phenomena that are common, but important to recognize and understand — such as the analysis of ventricular extrastimuli on ventriculoatrial conduction — are provided to lay the groundwork for interpreting more complex findings. Subsequent illustrations cover a spectrum of supraventricular and ventricular arrhythmias. The importance of a careful systematic approach well grounded in the fundamentals is illustrated in the final example in Section 9 discussed by Dr George J Klein, one of the leading thinkers in clinical cardiac electrophysiology.

This text will be valuable to everyone in the electrophysiology laboratory: technicians, fellows in training and experienced electrophysiologists.

William G Stevenson
Brigham and Women's Hospital, Boston, MA, USA

ABBREVIATIONS AND CONVENTIONS USED IN THIS BOOK

Abbreviations are given where they first occur in the text and in the figure legends, but a list is also given below for reference. The following conventions — labeling of electrograms in the tracings — are used throughout (with one or two exceptions, detailed where they occur):

CS	coronary sinus
HRA	high right atrium
HBE	His bundle electrogram
Map	mapping/ablation catheter
RV	right ventricle (usually apex)
Uni	unipolar electrogram (from mapping catheter)

Where two electrode pairs from the same catheter appear, they are labeled D (distal) and P (proximal), and where multiple electrode pairs appear, they are labeled numerically, starting from the distal end. Thus DCS and PCS indicate distal and proximal coronary sinus; HBE D and HBE P are the distal and proximal electrode pairs of a quadripolar His bundle catheter; and CS 1–2 and CS 9–10 are the distal and proximal electrode pairs from a decapolar coronary sinus electrode.

All of the tracings in this book come from computerized data acquisition equipment, most commonly output on a laser printer at 100 mm/s, but scaled down to fit the page size here. Other than where indicated, the time scale is indicated by large marks at the top and bottom of each tracing indicating 1 second (e.g. Tracing 1.3), or by large, medium and small graduations indicating 1000, 100 and 10 ms (e.g. Tracings 1.4b).

Abbreviations

AF	atrial fibrillation
AP	accessory pathway
AV	atrioventricular
AVN	atrioventricular node
AVNRT	AV nodal reentrant tachycardia
AVRT	AV reentrant tachycardia
BCL	basic cycle length
CL	cycle length
CS	coronary sinus
CSNRT	corrected sinus node recovery time
DC	direct current
ERP	effective refractory period
FP	fast pathway
FRP	functional refractory period
HBE	His bundle electrogram
HRA	high right atrium
ICD	implantable cardioverter defibrillator
IVC	inferior vena cava
JET	junctional ectopic tachycardia
LAO	left anterior oblique
LRA	low right atrium
LV	left ventricle
LVOT	left ventricular outflow tract
PAC	premature atrial contraction
PEI	pre-excitation index
PJRT	permanent junctional reciprocating tachycardia
PPI	post-pacing interval
Purk	Purkinje
PVC	premature ventricular contraction

RA	right atrium
RAO	right anterior oblique
RBB	right bundle branch
RBBB	right bundle branch block
RF	radiofrequency
RRP	relative refractory period
RV	right ventricle
RVA	right ventricular apex
RVOT	right ventricular outflow tract
SACT	sino-atrial conduction time
SCL	sinus cycle length
SNRT	sinus node recovery time
SP	slow pathway
SR	sinus rhythm
SVT	supraventricular tachycardia
TCL	tachycardia cycle length
TRT	total recovery time
Uni	unipolar electrogram
VA	ventriculoatrial
VF	ventricular fibrillation
VT	ventricular tachycardia
WCL	Wenckebach cycle length

Cardiac electrophysiology (EP) is a highly specialized branch of clinical cardiology with particular requirements in terms of facilities, staffing and expertise. Most of this book is concerned with arrhythmia mechanisms and the practical detail of cardiac EP procedures: this introductory section is intended to provide background information.

The equipment required for fluoroscopy and general patient care during EP procedures is outlined first — most of this is to be found in any modern cardiac catheterization laboratory. The responsibilities of the staff in an EP laboratory are then discussed. The emphasis then moves to patient preparation and general care for an EP procedure, including informed consent, monitoring and sedation/anesthesia. Next, the selection and placement of catheters for a routine diagnostic EP study is outlined. Finally, the specialized equipment used in an EP laboratory for cardiac stimulation and the amplification, filtering and recording of intracardiac signals is discussed.

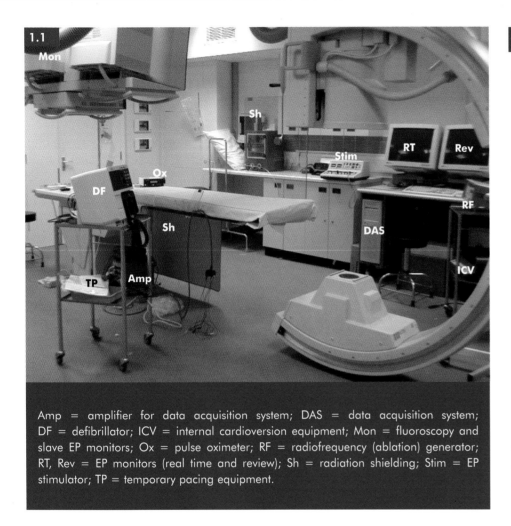

1.1

Mon
Sh
RT
Rev
Stim
Ox
DF
RF
Sh
DAS
ICV
TP
Amp

Amp = amplifier for data acquisition system; DAS = data acquisition system; DF = defibrillator; ICV = internal cardioversion equipment; Mon = fluoroscopy and slave EP monitors; Ox = pulse oximeter; RF = radiofrequency (ablation) generator; RT, Rev = EP monitors (real time and review); Sh = radiation shielding; Stim = EP stimulator; TP = temporary pacing equipment.

A laboratory used for EP and pacing procedures is shown in Figure 1.1. The C-arm fluoroscopy and radiographic table can be seen in addition to the labeled equipment.

1.1A EQUIPMENT

- The *radiographic table* on which the patient is placed is movable to allow panning. It may also permit a degree of head-down tilt to assist with both subclavian/jugular venipuncture and the management of hypotension. Some EP laboratories double-up as a facility for tilt-testing, in which case the table allows up to 90° of head-up tilt.
- The *image intensifier* permits left and right oblique fluoroscopic projections, and preferably also allows cranial and caudal tilt. For the purpose of diagnostic EP studies, a simple image intensifier may suffice to allow catheter placement. However, for complex ablation procedures that may require prolonged fluoroscopy, modern fixed-arm equipment is best; this allows digital image acquisition and provides optimum shielding, reduced scatter and pulsed fluoroscopy to reduce exposure for patients and staff. All staff are issued with appropriate protective clothing and radiation dosimeters. Staff movement is limited during the procedure, therefore extra shields that are not excessively intrusive can be used to reduce exposure.
- *Specialized EP equipment*: cardiac stimulator and data acquisition/monitoring system (see Section 1.4); a range of diagnostic and mapping/ablation catheters (see Section 1.3); radiofrequency (RF) energy generator (see Section 8.1); possibly equipment allowing alternative methods for mapping and ablation (see Section 8.8) and for low energy internal cardioversion.
- *Pulse oximetry* for monitoring respiration in the sedated patient.
- *Hemodynamic monitoring equipment*: automated non-invasive blood pressure equipment and/or transducers for invasive monitoring.
- An *intravenous infusion pump* and a range of *intravenous (IV) fluids and drugs*, including: sedative and analgesic agents; antiemetics; antihistamines and corticosteroids; and electrophysiologically active drugs (antiarrhythmics, isoproterenol, atropine and adenosine).
- An *external defibrillator*, suitable for use with standard paddles and remote defibrillation pads.

- A *temporary pacemaker,* as back up for the cardiac stimulator, and in case a patient needs to be transferred out of the EP laboratory while still pacing-dependent.
- *Resuscitation equipment* (e.g. airways, endotracheal tubes, oxygen, suction, emergency drugs).

In addition to the above, certain other emergency facilities should be within easy reach, though not necessarily in the EP laboratory itself, to cover for rare eventualities. These include echocardiography, a pericardial aspiration set and full anesthetic and intensive care facilities. Most EP procedures are performed within major cardiac centers where percutaneous coronary intervention and cardiac surgery also take place. However, it is exceptionally rare for an EP procedure (properly planned with careful risk assessment) to give rise to the need for these interventions.

1.1B   STAFFING

EP procedures are performed by a specialized team, whose composition varies between centers but which fulfills the following tasks:

- Invasive tasks (insertion of percutaneous sheaths, positioning of intracardiac electrode catheters and manipulation of mapping catheters).
- Operation of EP equipment (the stimulator, the data acquisition system and the ablation generator).
- Direct care of patient (e.g. nursing care; monitoring hemodynamic status, airway, oxygen saturation; and administration of oxygen, IV drugs and sometimes general anesthesia).

In a teaching center, it is common for a trainee to perform invasive tasks, while the electrophysiologist observes and directs the procedure ('scrubbing in' only for difficult or high-risk cases). The electrophysiologist, a technician or a second trainee may operate the stimulator and recording equipment. Administration of IV drugs and general patient care are the responsibility of a nurse (who may have specialist training in conscious sedation) and/or an anesthetist; this person may also operate the defibrillator where necessary.

In a private institution, the electrophysiologist typically handles the catheters and may operate the ablation generator using a pedal. He/she directs a technician who operates the stimulator and recording equipment and adjusts the ablation generator settings. Again, general patient care and drug administration are the responsibility of a nurse and/or anesthetist.

Movement of the table and positioning of the fluoroscopy equipment is generally performed by the catheter operator or other staff present. However, the presence of a radiographer is helpful and may be a legal requirement in some countries.

Specific training requirements for the medical and non-medical staff in an EP laboratory vary between countries and are constantly evolving (see Further Reading). It goes without saying that the EP team should be capable of basic resuscitation, and that a fully equipped and trained resuscitation team should be on site.

1.2 PATIENT PREPARATION

1.2A INFORMED CONSENT

The purpose and benefits of the EP procedure are explained to the patient and their family; they are also advised of the potential complications. The latter can be divided into four categories:

(i) *Vascular complications* common to all invasive cardiac procedures — approximately 1–5% of patients develop marked bruising or the formation of palpable hematomas. More serious complications (venous thrombosis, arterial occlusion, formation of fistulae or false aneurysms) follow <1% of procedures.

(ii) *Major but treatable complications* of invasive cardiac procedures, especially pneumothorax and cardiac tamponade — these complications should not occur in much more than 1% of cases, and if quickly recognized and competently treated should not result in any permanent after-effects.

(iii) *Specific complications* of EP procedures — patients should be warned that certain EP procedures carry particular risks:

- *AV nodal damage requiring permanent pacemaker implantation* — 'slow pathway' ablation for AV nodal reentry carries a small risk (around 1%) of permanent AV nodal damage, though this may be higher or lower according to the aggressiveness of the approach (see Section 8.3). Catheter ablation of accessory pathways anywhere along the septal portion of the tricuspid annulus (see Section 8.5) carries a 2–3% risk of AV nodal damage. It is important to discuss these risks in detail with patients, so that, once the diagnostic part of the procedure is complete, the operator can be clear on how to proceed. For example, for many individuals it may be appropriate to attempt ablation of an accessory pathway in a low risk area but not one near the AV node.

- *Arrhythmia induction* — atrial fibrillation may complicate up to 10% of EP studies for supraventricular tachycardia. While the arrhythmia is usually self-terminating, if sustained it may prevent completion of the procedure, and cardioversion may therefore be necessary. Sustained ventricular tachycardia (VT) or ventricular fibrillation is very rare during EP procedures for supraventricular arrhythmias, but quite common when programmed ventricular stimulation is performed (see Section 7.1).

- *Thromboembolic complications* — extensive RF ablation procedures in the left atrium (such as linear ablation) using currently available technology carry a significant risk of thromboembolism, and RF ablation within the pulmonary veins may cause irreversible stenosis leading to pulmonary hypertension.

(iv) *Life-threatening, irreversible complications* — EP studies and catheter ablation of supraventricular tachycardias, if carefully performed by appropriately trained practitioners, are among the safest invasive cardiac procedures. The risk of death, myocardial infarction or stroke is up to 0.5% overall, and is highest in patients with structural heart disease, multiple ablation targets and in the elderly. This risk should be considerably lower with routine catheter ablation for supraventricular tachycardias. Systemic thromboembolism and coronary artery trauma are obviously largely confined to left-sided procedures. Proper training and a meticulous approach to detail (e.g. anticoagulation, care in crossing the aortic valve, avoidance of air emboli) are needed to ensure that the risk of these major complications remains very small indeed. Patients should also be advised of the small but definite risk of adverse effects related to radiation exposure.

1.2B GENERAL CARE OF THE PATIENT UNDERGOING EP PROCEDURES

Patient preparation

Antiarrhythmic drugs should where possible be discontinued for at least four half-lives (for most drugs, 2–3 days) prior to any EP procedure, with the possible exception of AV node ablation. Amiodarone presents a particular problem in this respect because of its long half-life. A case-by-case decision regarding discontinuation of drugs is required for those patients either on amiodarone or with severe arrhythmic symptoms off drugs. As with any invasive procedure, anticoagulant drugs should be discontinued, and hypoglycemic drug regimens may need to be adjusted or interrupted.

EP procedures are always performed after a suitable period of fasting (at least 6 hours, and usually overnight). Due to the consequent dehydration, patients may tolerate sustained tachycardias poorly and an IV fluid infusion may be beneficial for prolonged procedures.

IV access should be obtained before the patient arrives in the EP laboratory, as vasovagal reactions are quite common during patient instrumentation.

Once the patient arrives in the EP laboratory, surface electrodes are attached to enable the acquisition of routine 12-lead ECGs (either by the EP recording system or a separate ECG recorder). A non-invasive blood pressure cuff is attached unless invasive monitoring is planned. Continuous pulse oximetry should also be performed if sedative drugs are to be given. Remote defibrillation pads may be attached if there is a significant chance that external shocks will be necessary, and are routine in many centers; these allow defibrillation to be performed with minimal disturbance and without interference to the sterile field. Finally, an indifferent skin electrode plate is placed if ablation is intended.

Sedation and anesthesia

Practice differs between EP units regarding the desirability of premedication, sedation and, indeed, anesthesia. Some hold that any medication may affect the inducibility of arrhythmias. Certainly these drugs may be avoided in unusual cases where arrhythmia non-inducibility is a known problem (e.g. normal heart VT, see Section 7.4). Our practice for most procedures is to give premedication and/or titrated conscious sedation using a combination of benzodiazepine and opiate drugs, combined with an antiemetic. General anesthesia is rarely necessary for electrophysiologic studies other than for psychological reasons (e.g. in young adults and children) or to permit external cardioversion.

1.3A ELECTRODE CATHETERS AND THEIR PLACEMENTS

Diagnostic electrode catheters (Figure 1.3a-i) are usually 5F or 6F, and carry at least two electrode pairs, to allow simultaneous pacing (via the distal pair, in contact with the endocardium) and recording (via the proximal pair), or to allow recording at more than one location. A selection of interelectrode spacing is available: 2-mm spacing provides signals registered over a very localized area, while greater electrode separation (5–10-mm) records signals reflecting a greater proportion of the chamber.

Figure 1.3a-i shows three types of diagnostic electrode catheter. Left: 2-mm spaced decapolar catheter for detailed recording of the His bundle and right bundle branch; middle: 2-8-2-mm spaced decapolar catheter for coronary sinus recording; right: 5-mm spaced quadripolar catheter for pacing and recording in the right atrium and ventricle.

Catheters for mapping and ablation are usually 7F or 8F, and are available with a variety of deflectable tip shapes (Figure 1.3a-ii and -iii). The most common types have a 4-mm tip, through which RF energy is delivered, and three ring electrodes.

Electrode catheters are almost always inserted using the Seldinger technique under local anesthesia. Some centers use the femoral veins exclusively, but access via the subclavian or jugular approach can be useful, especially for coronary sinus cannulation. The median basilic vein is also occasionally used.

Figure 1.3a-ii shows a deflectable 4-mm mapping/ablation catheter with a small curve.

Figure 1.3a-iii shows a deflectable 4-mm mapping/ablation catheter with an extended reach.

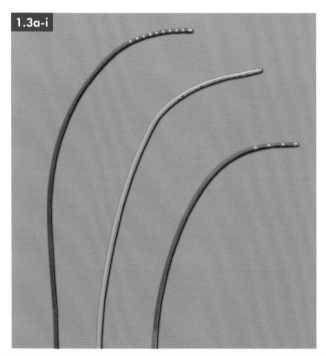
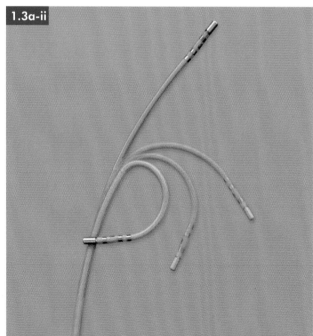
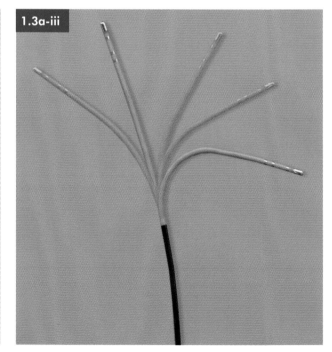

1.3B STANDARD CATHETER ELECTRODES

A standard diagnostic EP study for the investigation of supraventricular tachycardia uses four catheter electrodes (Figure 1.3b):

High right atrium
A shaped quadripolar catheter (e.g. 'Josephson' type) with 5-5-5-mm spacing is advanced from a femoral vein and placed in contact with the right atrial wall. Ideally, the tip should be on the lateral wall, near the superior vena cava/right atrial junction.

Right ventricular apex
A quadripolar catheter with 5- or 10-mm spacing is advanced from a femoral vein and placed with the tip as close as possible to the right ventricular apex.

The exact positions of the right atrial and right ventricular electrodes may have to be adjusted to achieve satisfactory sensing and pacing.

Coronary sinus
The coronary sinus is usefully situated along the mitral annulus, allowing registration of electrograms from the left atrium and ventricle without the need for arterial puncture. A range of multipolar catheters is available for coronary sinus recording. Anatomic variation requires some flexibility of approach. Access is usually easiest entering the heart via the superior vena cava, after subclavian or jugular venipuncture, but the femoral approach is usually successful if a steerable catheter is used. We prefer to use decapolar catheters with 2-8-2-8-2-8-2-8-2-mm spacing which results in five closely spaced bipoles 1 cm apart. This allows recording of sharp electrograms over a large portion of the coronary sinus. If possible, the catheter is placed so that its proximal bipole overlies the lateral border of the vertebral bodies in the posteroanterior projection: this generally approximates to the location of the coronary sinus os, but more importantly is a reproducible landmark.

His bundle
The His bundle catheter is used to record electrograms in the region of the atrioventricular (AV) node. It is usually advanced from a femoral vein to a position straddling the tricuspid annulus in its superior portion. At the correct location, a clear His bundle electrogram is seen between atrial and ventricular electrograms. Direct recording of AV nodal activation is not possible in clinical practice, but the His bundle catheter indicates the timing of impulses entering and leaving the AV node via the adjacent atrial tissue and the His bundle, or vice versa. We usually use a curved-tip or steerable quadripolar catheter with 2-2-2-mm electrode spacing, giving 'distal His' and 'proximal His' electrograms. For detailed His bundle recording (e.g. to document antidromic tachycardia, see Section 6.8), a closely spaced multipolar catheter may be useful.

Other electrode catheters
The above diagnostic electrodes usually suffice for the purpose of routine diagnostic EP studies and catheter ablation. More specialized catheters are described in the relevant sections of this book.

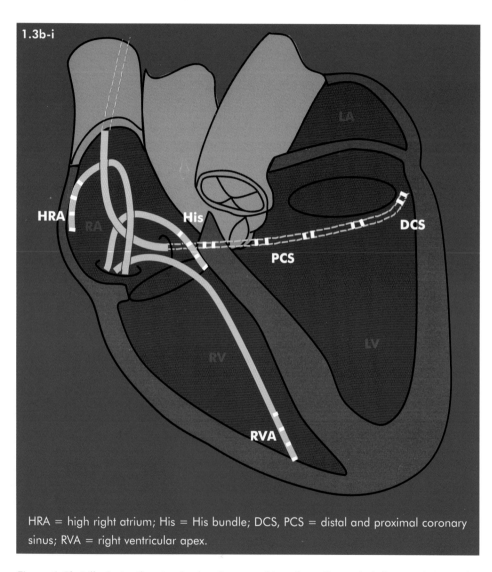

1.3b-i

HRA = high right atrium; His = His bundle; DCS, PCS = distal and proximal coronary sinus; RVA = right ventricular apex.

Figure 1.3b-i illustrates the standard catheter positions for a 'four-wire' diagnostic EP study.

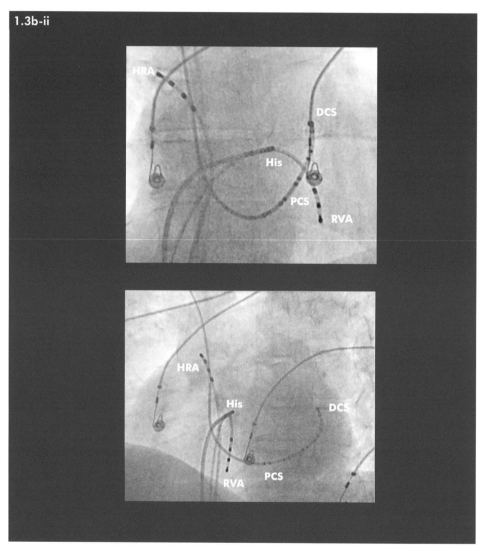

1.3b-ii

Figure 1.3b-ii shows the catheter positions for a standard 'four-wire' diagnostic EP study in the posteroanterior (top) and left anterior oblique (bottom) fluoroscopic projections. Abbreviations as in Figure 1.3b-i.

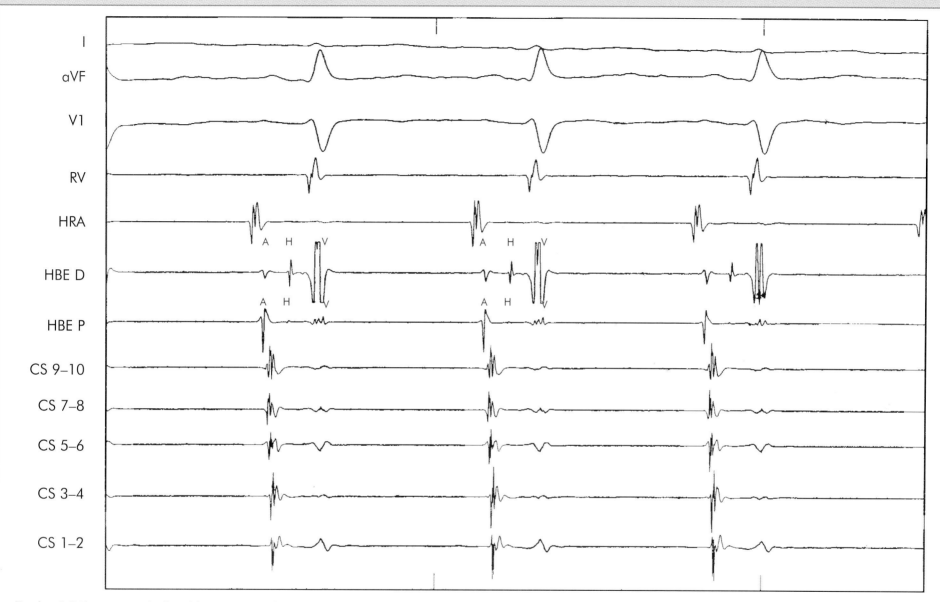

Tracing 1.3 Electrograms displayed during standard four-wire study in sinus rhythm. Although all twelve surface ECG leads are recorded, only three approximately orthogonal leads are shown, for clarity. The right ventricular apex (RV) and high right atrium (HRA) leads show sharp single chamber electrograms. The His bundle catheter records activity adjacent to the AV node; the distal bipole (HBE D) favoring the His bundle electrogram (H) and the adjacent ventricular myocardium (V), while the proximal bipole (HBE P) shows a large atrial electrogram (A). Note that, although the ventricular spike recorded by the His bundle comes from tissue adjacent to the bundle of His, the earliest ventricular activity is at the apex (RV). The electrograms recorded by the bipoles of the decapolar coronary sinus catheter are labeled CS 9–10 (proximal) to CS 1–2 (distal); each shows a sharp atrial electrogram followed by a smaller ventricular electrogram.

A standard set-up for patient stimulation, digital electrophysiological monitoring and RF ablation is shown diagrammatically in Figure 1.4a.

1.4A   THE STIMULATOR

The stimulator, which may be separate or integral to the EP monitoring system, is capable of delivering constant current pacing impulses. With satisfactory positioning of the catheter electrodes, current thresholds under 3 mA for the atrium and 2 mA for the ventricle can usually be achieved with a 2 ms pulse width. Higher thresholds may have to be accepted in some circumstances, for example where the myocardium is diseased, if pacing in unusual locations (e.g. the coronary sinus) or in the presence of antiarrhythmic drugs. The stimulator output is conventionally set at twice the measured diastolic threshold for each location.

The stimulator is capable of a variety of modes: simple pacing (inhibited or fixed); rapid pacing (at rates of 300 bpm and over); delivery of single and multiple timed extrastimuli following sensed beats (sinus rhythm or tachycardia); and delivery of extrastimuli following a paced drive train. These stimulation modes are described in Section 2. Many stimulators are capable of output through more than one channel, though the equivalent of dual chamber pacing is rarely required in routine EP procedures.

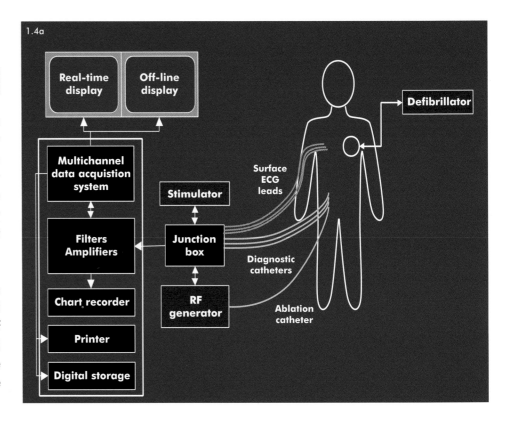

1.4B   AMPLIFICATION AND FILTERING

The physiological signals acquired via surface and intracardiac electrodes are typically <10 mV in amplitude, and therefore require considerable amplification before they can be digitized, displayed and stored. The avoidance of extraneous signals at the input stage of the amplifier is essential: all electrical equipment should be checked to avoid current leakages, and should be properly earthed and shielded. Careful attention must also be paid to skin preparation for surface electrodes. When setting up a new EP laboratory, it may take considerable time to track down sources of noise, but this time is well invested.

Filters (nowadays, generally digital) are used to eliminate unwanted components of a signal. Three types of filter may be used:

(i) *High-pass* filters eliminate components below a given frequency. In the surface ECG, components such as the T-wave are of relatively low frequency, and high-pass filtering around 0.05 Hz is used to preserve these components while eliminating baseline drift. On the other hand, with the intracardiac electrogram, high frequency components are of the most interest (electrophysiologists are essentially concerned with the timing of these signals rather than their true morphologies), and high-pass filtering of 30–50 Hz is used to eliminate the low frequency components.

One exception to this rule is the unipolar electrogram, which is used during catheter activation mapping (see Section 8.4B): the polarity of the signal reflects the direction of myocardial activation, and the signal morphology (and therefore low frequency components) must be preserved. Unipolar electrograms usually go through a high-pass filter of 0.05 Hz, or none at all.

(ii) *Low-pass* filters eliminate components above a given frequency. There are essentially no intracardiac signals of interest much above 300 Hz. To eliminate

noise at higher frequencies, low-pass filters are generally set to around 500 Hz for intracardiac signals or 200 Hz for surface electrocardiography.

(iii) *Notch filters* eliminate signals at a specific frequency. The most common notch filters are set up to eliminate mains interference, i.e. 50 Hz in Europe and 60 Hz in North America. Since these frequencies are an important component of intracardiac signals, notch filters inevitably cause a degree of distortion.

It is important to recognize the effect of filtering on physiological signals in order to avoid misinterpretation. This is illustrated in Tracings 1.4b-i and –ii.

1.4C   DISPLAY, STORAGE AND PRINTING

After amplification, signals are digitized and filtered by a computerized data acquisition system. This system writes the data to a hard disk and/or optical drive, at the same time as displaying signals on a cathode ray tube. The ideal system provides a versatile choice of display configurations; a wide range of sweep speeds (up to 200 mm/s); triggered sweeps; and the ability to turn each channel on and off, and adjust its size and other characteristics. In addition to the real-time display, a second monitor providing off-line analysis including multiple cursors for accurate measurement of intervals is invaluable. Some systems are also able to perform automated interval measurements; provide a case report; and incorporate other signals such as fluoroscopic images. All modern systems use laser printers to provide paper copies of tracings (all of the tracings in this book are derived from these). Some systems can also provide an analog high-definition continuous paper trace using an inkjet (e.g. Siemens Mingograf) or thermal paper printer. Many electrophysiologists believe that these 'old-fashioned' chart recorders reproduce intracardiac signals better than laser printers.

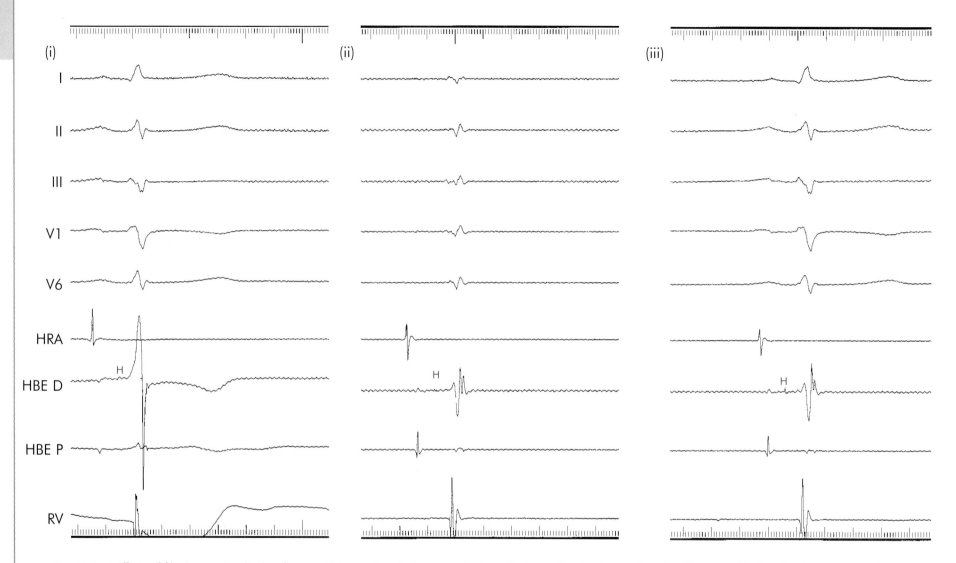

Tracing 1.4b-i Effects of filtering on standard surface and intracardiac electrograms. An imperfect recording has been selected, with a small His bundle electrogram and some mains interference ('hum'), which is most obvious in the most highly amplified channels (e.g. HBE D). Left: all channels are filtered with a high-pass of 0.05 Hz and a low-pass of 400 Hz. The surface ECG is acceptable, but the intracardiac electrograms contain low frequency components that are clinically irrelevant and obscure the important high frequency components. Center: all channels are now filtered with a high-pass of 30 Hz, removing low frequency components. The intracardiac electrograms are now more acceptable, but the QRS morphologies on the surface ECG are altered, and the P- and T-waves, which are entirely low frequency signals, are eliminated. Right: typical normal settings, with the surface ECG filtered at 0.05–200 Hz, avoiding distortion of the signal morphologies, while intracardiac signals are filtered at 30–400 Hz, removing the low frequency components.

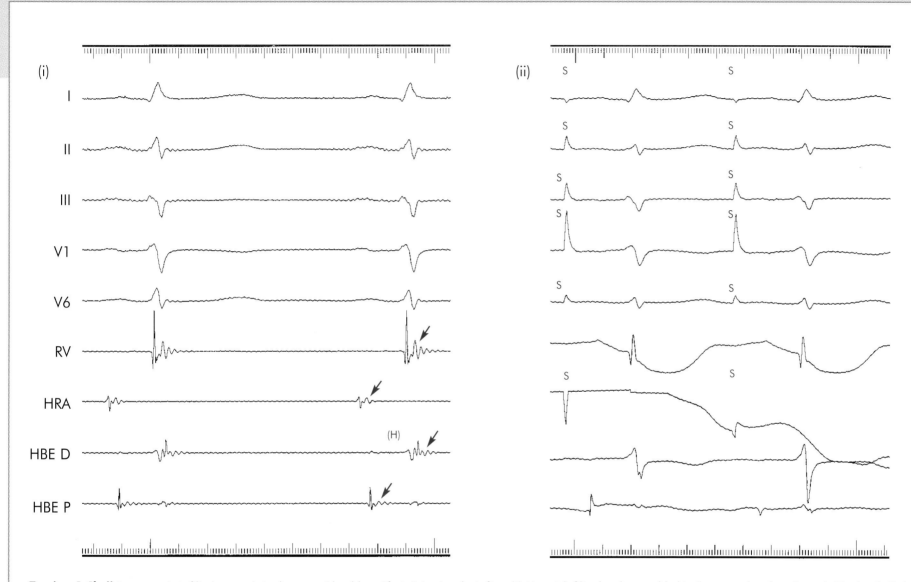

Tracing 1.4b-ii Inappropriate filtering can introduce considerable artifacts into signals. Left: a 60 Hz notch filter has been added to the normal settings (seen in Tracing 1.4b-i, right). The 'hum' due to mains interference is reduced, but the His bundle spike is eliminated, and each of the intracardiac signals is distorted by 'ringing' following its high frequency components (arrowed). Right: elimination of high frequency components with a 20 Hz low-pass filter makes atrial pacing spikes (S) resemble electrograms.

These tracings illustrate the principle that the best signals are obtained by careful patient instrumentation and elimination of sources of noise, rather than trying to correct for deficiencies by electronic means.

FURTHER READING

1. Electrophysiologic investigation: technical aspects. In: Josephson ME. Clinical Cardiac Electrophysiology, Second Edition. Philadelphia/London: Lea and Febiger, 1993:5–12.

2. Adams DE. Organization of the interventional laboratory. In: Singer I, editor. Interventional Electrophysiology. Baltimore: Williams and Wilkins, 1997:3–25.

3. Techniques in electrophysiologic testing. In: Prystowsky EN, Klein GJ. Cardiac Arrhythmias: An Integrated Approach for the Clinician. New York: McGraw-Hill, 1994:299–334.

4. Calkins H, Yong P, Miller JM et al. Catheter ablation of accessory pathways, atrioventricular nodal reentrant tachycardia, and the atrioventricular junction: final results of a prospective, multicenter clinical trial. The Atakr Multicenter Investigators Group. Circulation 1999;99(2):262–70.

5. Guidelines for Clinical Intracardiac Electrophysiological and Catheter Ablation Procedures. A report of the American College of Cardiology/American Heart Association Task Force on practice guidelines. (Committee on Clinical Intracardiac Electrophysiologic and Catheter Ablation Procedures). Developed in collaboration with the North American Society of Pacing and Electrophysiology. Circulation 1995;92(3):673–91.

After patient preparation, catheter placement and threshold testing, a routine electrophysiology (EP) study commences with measurement of the spontaneous sinus rate and intracardiac conduction intervals. Tests of sinus node function may be performed as part of a complete EP study, but are often dispensed with if sinus node dysfunction is not a suspected diagnosis.

Two kinds of pacing technique are then used to provide functional testing: extrastimulus testing and incremental pacing.

Extrastimulus testing is used to observe and measure refractory periods and dynamic changes in conduction accompanying sudden changes in cycle length.

Incremental pacing (overdriving the spontaneous rhythm) allows the observation and measurement of impulse conduction and tissue refractoriness during (quasi-) steady-state conditions, and the recovery of normal function after the cessation of pacing.

2.1A   RHYTHM AND CYCLE LENGTH

Basic intervals should be measured during sinus rhythm — if this is not possible, the rhythm should be stated.

Some conduction intervals, especially the AH interval, vary significantly with heart rate, and especially with the preceding cycle length. It follows that measurements should be made during a period of stable heart rate, and that the cycle length immediately preceding the complex to be measured is recorded.

Figure 2.1a indicates the structures reflected in each basic interval measurement.

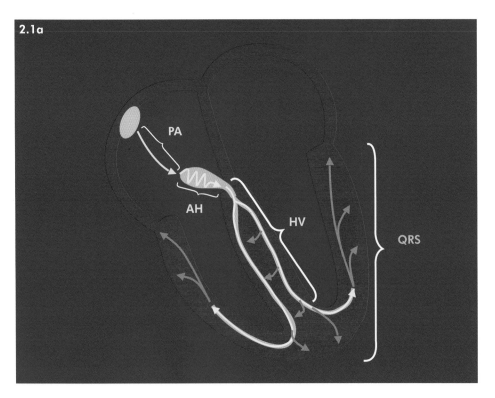

2.1a

2.1B   THE PA INTERVAL

The PA interval is the time taken for activation to travel between two fairly fixed points in the right atrium — the earliest atrial activation in the region of the sinus node and the region of the atrioventricular node. A prolonged PA interval indicates delay in intra-atrial conduction, usually due to atrial disease or drugs.

The PA interval is measured between the earliest recorded atrial activity in any channel (either the P-wave onset, or that of the earliest atrial electrogram) and the rapid deflection of the atrial electrogram on the His bundle catheter.

The earliest atrial activation is almost always the beginning of the surface P-wave, and the timing of the atrial electrogram is taken from the 'intrinsic' deflection (the first high-frequency component of the electrogram, which represents local rather than far-field activity). A PA interval of 25–55 ms is considered normal.[†]

[†]The 'normal' values for conduction intervals given in this section apply to adults only (and should not be considered as set in stone). Various authors have published differing reference ranges, but these are usually within 10 ms of the values given here.

2.1C THE AH INTERVAL

The AH interval is the time taken for the cardiac impulse to travel over the atrioventricular (AV) node, and is measured from the electrograms recorded by the His bundle catheter. AV nodal activation cannot be directly recorded by conventional techniques, but the AH interval is measured as the time taken from arrival of the signal at the atrium adjacent to the node to its emergence at the His bundle.

The AH interval is measured between the atrial electrogram recorded by the His bundle catheter and the beginning of the His electrogram itself.

As before, the timing of the atrial electrogram is taken from its intrinsic deflection. However, the timing of the His electrogram is taken from its earliest onset, as this represents the time the impulse arrives at the His bundle. An AH interval of 55–125 ms is considered normal.

The AH interval, reflecting conduction time in the AV node, is susceptible to modulation by a number of factors, especially autonomic tone. It is quite common for the well-sedated patient in the EP laboratory to have a prolonged AH interval because of enhanced vagal tone. If confirmation is required that this is the case, atropine can be given. Conduction in the AV node also varies with cycle length, due to its decremental properties (see Section 2.3A).

2.1D THE DURATION OF THE HIS BUNDLE ELECTROGRAM

The duration of the His bundle electrogram is an estimate of the total time taken for activation of the His bundle. It is not routinely measured.

The His bundle electrogram (HBE) duration is the time from the beginning of the very first component of the HBE to the end of its very last component.

Measured with a 10 mm spaced bipolar catheter electrode, the HBE duration corresponds to the total conduction time through the His bundle, and should be <30 ms. Minor conduction delay within the His bundle is manifest by a notched or fragmented deflection and is not sufficient to cause significant prolongation of the PR interval. More significant delay is unusual, but can cause a 'split' HBE with separate early and late components.

2.1E   THE HV INTERVAL

The HV interval is the time taken for conduction over the specialized fibers of the His-Purkinje system.

The HV interval is measured between the His bundle electrogram and the earliest recorded ventricular activation.

As with the AH interval, the timing of the His electrogram is taken from its onset. The earliest recorded ventricular activation is almost always the beginning of the surface QRS complex. An HV interval of 35–55 ms is considered normal.

Together, the PA, AH and HV intervals indicate what proportions of the PR interval can be ascribed to conduction in the atrium, AV node and His-Purkinje system.

2.1F   QRS DURATION AND THE QT INTERVAL

The duration of the QRS complex indicates the duration of ventricular activation and the QT interval represents the combination of ventricular activation and repolarization. These intervals are both measured from the surface ECG. As the QT varies greatly with heart rate, it is often expressed as a corrected value, QTc.

A number of formulae exist for the derivation of QTc, of which the most widely accepted is that of Bazett:

$$QTc = QT/\sqrt{RR}^{\dagger}$$

A QRS duration ≤100 ms is considered normal, though hemiblock can be diagnosed on morphological grounds with a QRS within this range. The upper limits of QTc are conventionally 440 ms for men and 460 ms for women, though some consider ranges of 430–450 ms and 450–470 ms, respectively, to be 'borderline'. Values above this are considered prolonged (though it is now clear that the long QT syndrome can often be present without clear QTc prolongation on the resting ECG).

Normal conduction intervals are listed on page 238.

†RR = mean RR interval, measured in seconds

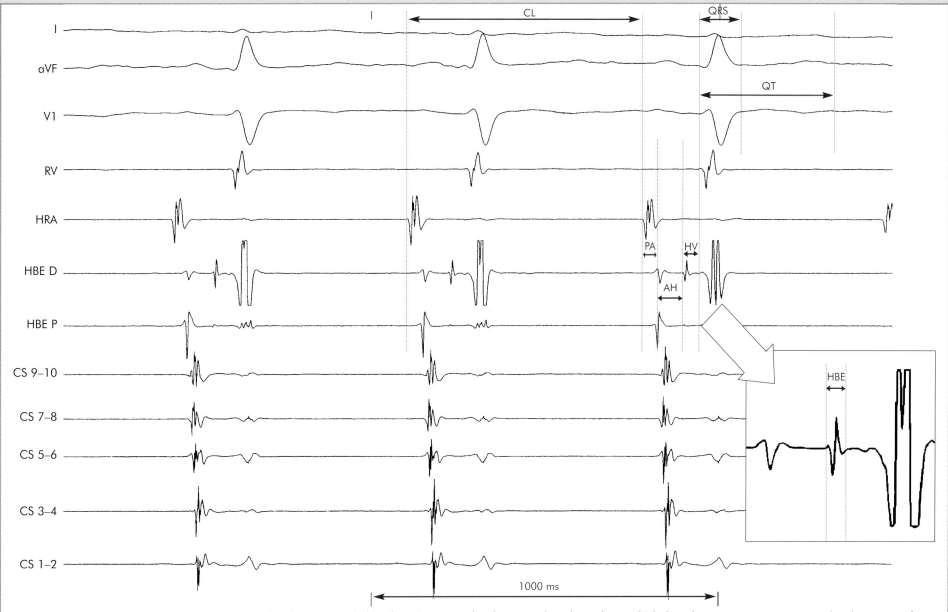

Tracing 2.1 Basic interval measurements. Note that the sinus cycle length (CL) measured is that preceding the cycle on which the other measurements are made. The timing of the atrial electrogram (PA and AH intervals) is taken from the intrinsic deflection (first sharp component). However, the timing of the His bundle electrogram (AH and HV intervals) is taken from its very first component. Measurement of the HBE duration is shown inset. In this instance, the following measurements were recorded (all in ms): cycle length (CL) = 673; PA = 46; AH = 73; HBE = 25; HV = 48; QRS = 105; QT = 401; QTc = 392. Note that, in this case, the PA interval was measured from the onset of the HRA electrogram: it is usually measured from the onset of the surface P-wave, as this is usually earlier.

Sinus node function testing may be of value in the investigation of a patient whose symptoms suggest a bradycardia. Two tests of sinus node function are in common use: the sinus node recovery time and the sino-atrial conduction time.

2.2A SINUS NODE RECOVERY TIME

As shown in Figure 2.2a, the sinus node recovery time (SNRT) is the time taken for sinus rhythm (yellow) to resume after a period (conventionally 30 s) of overdrive atrial pacing (blue). A certain amount of time is taken for paced impulses to invade the sinus node and for sinus impulses to escape, thus the SNRT that is measured overestimates the true time taken for sinus nodal tissue to recover (indicated by asterisk in figure).

The sinus node recovery time (SNRT) is the interval measured in the high right atrium (HRA) from the last paced complex to the first spontaneous complex after the cessation of pacing.

The SNRT varies with the sinus rate, so the corrected sinus node recovery time is a more useful measure.

The corrected sinus node recovery time (CSNRT) is the sinus node recovery time minus the sinus cycle length (SCL).

When sinus rhythm resumes after pacing, the first cycles are usually a little longer than the basic sinus cycle length, and the total recovery time reflects this phenomenon.

The total recovery time (TRT) is the interval between the cessation of pacing and the return to the basic sinus cycle length.

The basic sinus cycle length should be measured during a period of stable rate, i.e. several beats after the resumption of sinus rhythm, or before the start of the pacing train. SNRT cannot be measured if the first atrial activity after the end of pacing arises elsewhere than the sinus node (as evaluated by the P-wave axis and atrial activation sequence).

Proper examination of sinus node recovery requires repeated measurements following pacing at several cycle lengths (e.g. twice each at 800, 700, 600, 500, 450, 400, 350 and possibly 300 ms). The longest values of SNRT and CSNRT obtained are used. Centers differ over what constitutes 'normal' sinus node recovery, but reasonable values would be: maximum SNRT <1500 ms, maximum CSNRT (undoubtedly the most useful measure) <550 ms and maximum TRT <5 s.

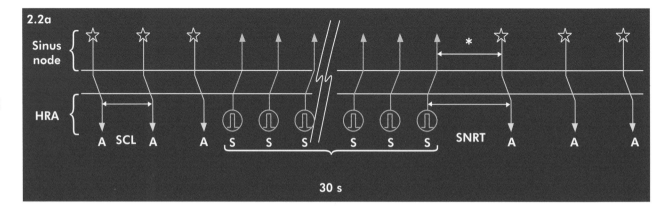

2.2a

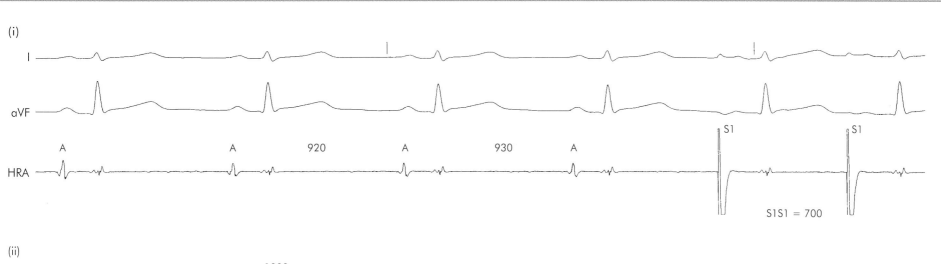

(i)

I

aVF

HRA

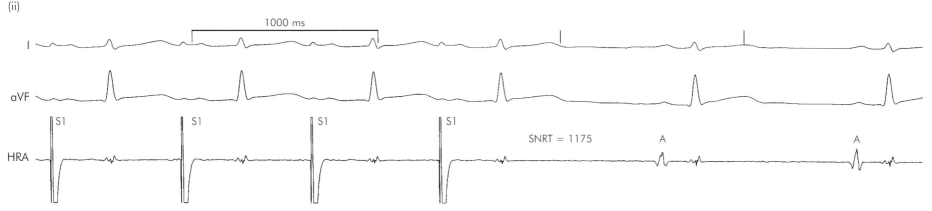

(ii)

I

1000 ms

aVF

HRA

Tracing 2.2a Surface ECG and high right atrial electrogram recorded during measurement of SNRTs. In 2.2a-i, the basic sinus cycle length just prior to the pacing train is approximately 925 ms. 2.2a-ii shows the end of the 30-second pacing train, and the resumption of sinus rhythm. The SNRT (last S1 to first A) is 1175 ms. The CSNRT on this occasion is therefore 250 ms.

2.2B SINO-ATRIAL CONDUCTION TIME

While the SNRT and CSNRT attempt to detect disease in the intrinsic function of the sinus node itself, the sino-atrial conduction time (SACT) is intended to detect delayed conduction between sinus node and adjacent atrial tissue. Calculation of the SACT is more complicated than that of the SNRT. The technique depends on resetting the sinus node with single extrastimuli delivered to the high right atrium.

In Figure 2.2b, sinus node impulses are represented in yellow and paced impulses in blue. It is assumed that the SACT, the interval taken for an impulse to travel between the sinus node and adjacent atrial tissue, is stable and equal in both inward and outward directions. During stable sinus rhythm, therefore, atrial cycles (A1) follow each sinus cycle after 1 x SACT. Thus the sinus cycle length (SCL) equals the atrial cycle length (A1A1).

Depending on the coupling interval of the extrastimulus (A1A2), one of a variety of responses can be seen:

(i) A late coupled atrial extrastimulus (long A1A2) collides with a sinus impulse outside the sinus node, and does not affect the timing of the next sinus beat (A3). Thus the return cycle length (A2A3) is a full compensatory pause, such that A1A2 + A2A3 = 2 x SCL.

(ii) An earlier coupled atrial extrastimulus (shorter A1A2) invades and resets the sinus node. The next sinus beat originates one SCL later, and is conducted out to the atrium. Thus A1A2 + A2A3 < 2 x SCL. Over a range of extrastimulus coupling intervals (A1A2), the return cycle length A2A3 does not vary greatly. During this range of coupling intervals, known as the 'zone of reset', the SACT can be calculated (see next page).

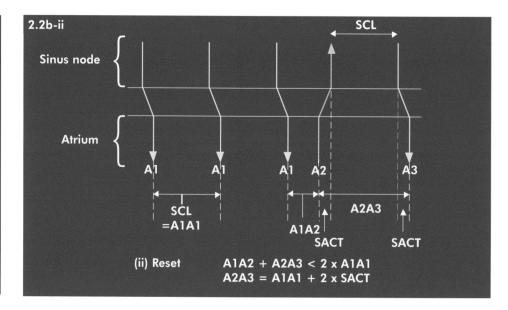

An earlier coupled atrial extrastimulus may evoke one of two responses:

(iii) If its conduction into the sinus node is blocked, the latter is not reset, and the next sinus impulse emerges on time. The extrastimulus is said to be 'interpolated' between sinus beats (perfect interpolation is rather unusual, as the escaping sinus beat is usually somewhat delayed).

(iv) The extrastimulus may give rise to local 'reentry', resulting in a very premature A3.

To calculate the SACT, atrial extrastimuli are delivered during sinus rhythm over a range of coupling intervals A1A2. It is important to allow several cycles between each extrastimulus so that sinus node automaticity is not suppressed. The zone of reset is identified as that range of A1A2 over which A2A3 does not vary, and SACT is given by:

$$\textbf{SACT} = \textbf{(A2A3 - A1A1) / 2}$$

Although there is some variation between normal ranges for SACT in different centers, most would accept values of a lower limit around 50 ms and an upper limit of 115 ms. These values are also consistent with measurements of the SACT made from direct recording.

A consistent measurement of the SACT can be difficult to obtain, and the predictive value of the test is rather questionable, so SACT is less frequently measured than the SNRT and CSNRT. Invasive tests should in any case be considered as an adjunct, rather than an alternative, to other techniques for detection of sinus node dysfunction such as ambulatory monitoring.

Normal sinus node function intervals are listed on page 238.

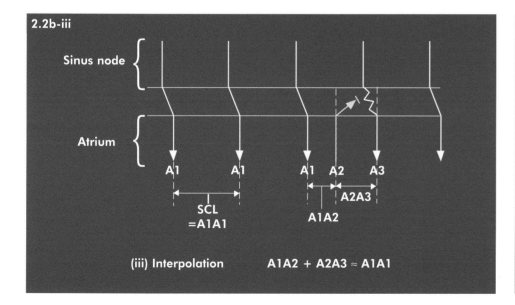

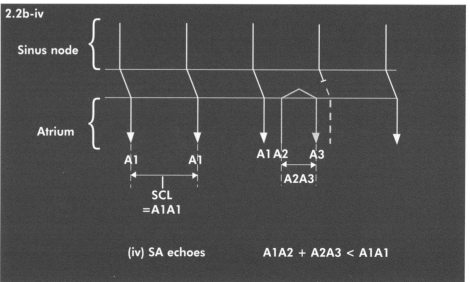

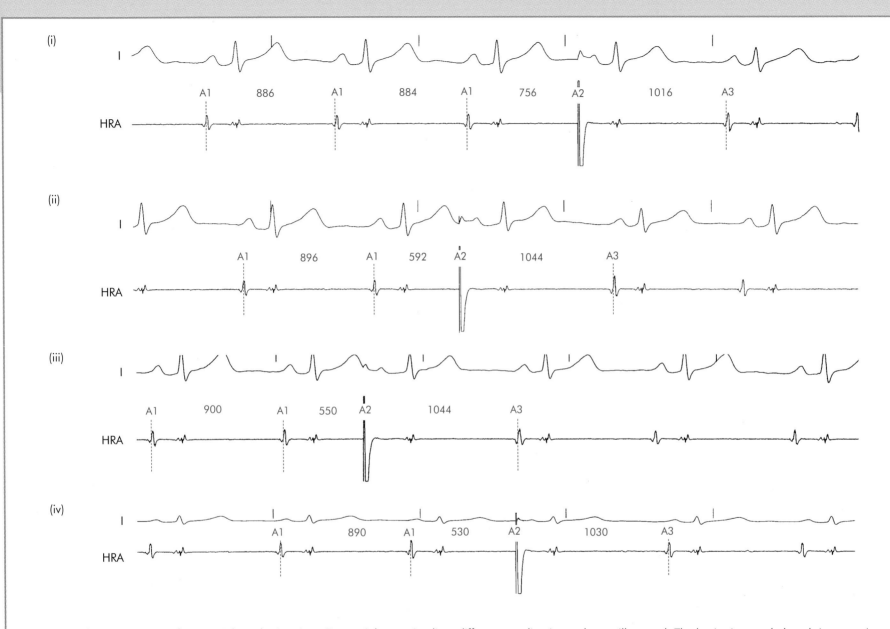

Tracing 2.2b Measurement of sino-atrial conduction time. Four atrial extrastimuli, at different coupling intervals, are illustrated. The basic sinus cycle length is approximately 890 ms throughout. In (i) the coupling interval is 756 ms and the return cycle A3 is 'on time' (A1A2 + A2A3 ≈ 2 x A1A1), indicating that the sinus node has not been reset (corresponding to Figure 2.2b-i). Tracings (ii)–(iv) are over a range of more closely coupled atrial extrastimuli (A1A2: 592, 550 and 530 ms), the return cycle A3 is 'early' (A1A2 + A2A3 < 2 x A1A1), but the return cycle length A2A3 is fairly constant (approximately 1040 ms). In this range, the sinus node is being reset (corresponding to Figure 2.2b-ii). The SACT is approximately (1040 - 890) / 2 = 75 ms.

A typical protocol for atrial extrastimulus testing uses a drive train of eight paced beats at a fixed cycle length (to establish a reasonable steady-state), followed by an extrastimulus delivered at the same site. The drive train is repeated while the coupling interval of the extrastimulus is progressively decreased until the atrium is no longer captured.

Several observations can be made during this form of stimulation. The most important of these are the dynamic properties of conduction over the AV node and the His-Purkinje system, as well as the refractory periods of the AV node and right atrium. Additionally, gross abnormalities of intra-atrial and sometimes intra-ventricular conduction may be demonstrated. The presence of dual AV nodal physiology (see Section 4) or abnormal conducting structures such as accessory pathways (see Section 5) may be demonstrated. Finally, extrastimulus testing may be used for arrhythmia induction (see Sections 3–6).

2.3A ANTEGRADE CONDUCTION OVER THE AV NODE

Atrial extrastimuli with long coupling intervals are conducted over the AV node at a fairly constant velocity (e.g. though this is dependent on the drive cycle length and autonomic tone). Thus in Figure 2.3a-i the AH intervals are the same following the extrastimuli (A2H2) as for cycles in the drive train (A1H1).

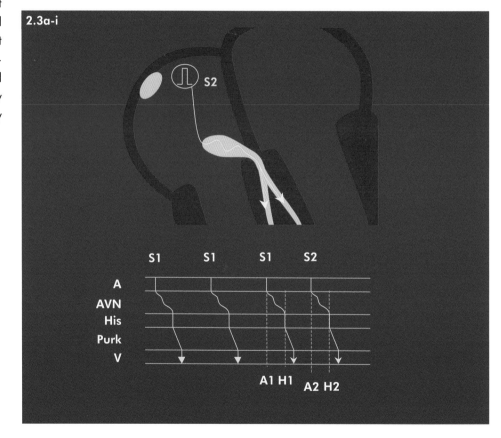

2.3a-i

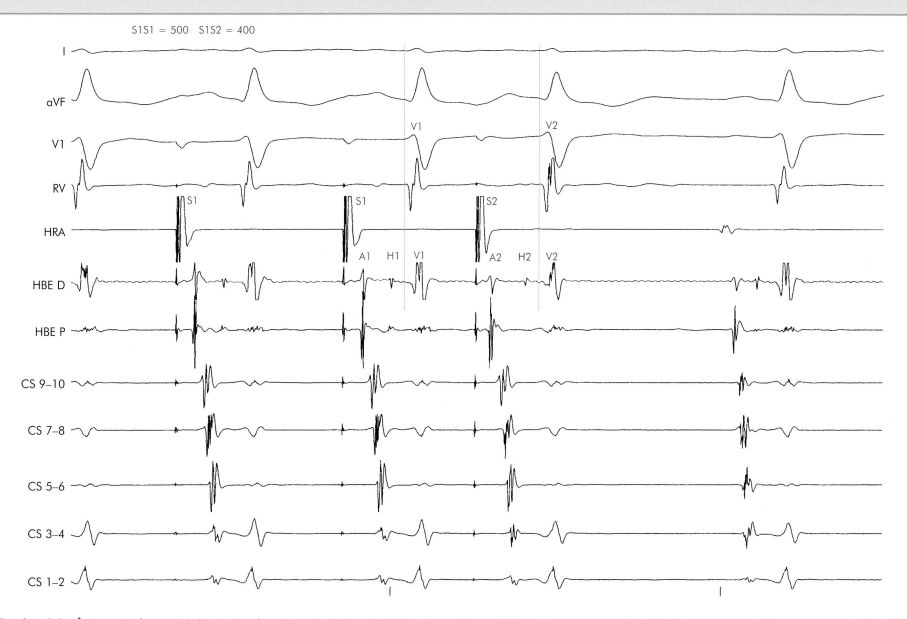

Tracing 2.3a-i The end of an atrial drive train of cycle length 500 ms (S1S1) is shown. The conduction time over the node (A1H1) is measured at 78 ms. An extrastimulus (S2) is delivered with a coupling interval of 400 ms (S1S2). The atrial impulse from the extrastimulus is conducted over the AV node slightly more slowly (A2H2 = 97 ms). There is no significant slowing of conduction either within the right atrium (S1A1 ≈ S2A2 ≈ 55 ms) or in the His-Purkinje system (H1V1 ≈ H2V2 ≈ 50 ms). Note that the timing of ventricular activation (cursors) is taken from the surface ECG, which precedes the ventricular deflection in the His bundle electrogram, as explained in Section 2.1.

With shorter coupling intervals, however, the conduction velocity through the AV node progressively decreases and the AH interval progressively lengthens (Figure 2.3a-ii). This phenomenon, known as 'decremental conduction', is of fundamental importance in clinical electrophysiology. It is a property of cardiac tissue (especially the AV node) that is principally dependent on a 'slow' inward calcium current for depolarization. The specialized conducting fibers of the His-Purkinje system are depolarized by 'fast' sodium channels ('phase 0' of the action potential), and their conduction velocity is virtually unchanged over a wide range of coupling intervals.[†] Atrial myocardial tissue does show some slowing in conduction with closely coupled extrastimuli, but this is usually far less than the AV node, and normal ventricular myocardium shows very little decremental conduction.

It should be noted that clinicians use the term 'decrement' to describe rate-dependent prolongation of conduction. To the basic scientist, the term is used to mean progressive loss of action potential strength as conduction progresses over a structure until it is insufficient to excite further tissue.

[†]This is the reason that Wenckebach-type AV conduction indicates block in the AV node, while sudden loss of conduction not preceded by slowing (Möbitz type II) suggests block in the His-Purkinje system.

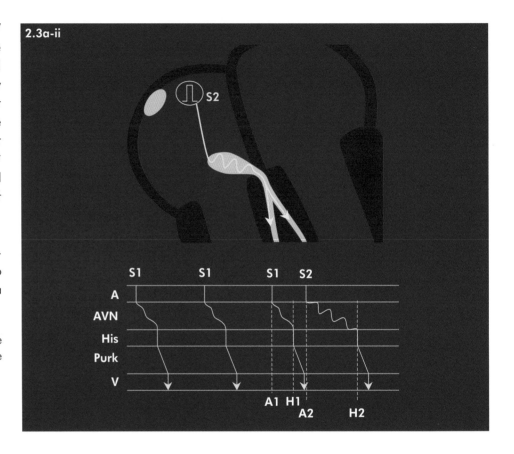

2.3a-ii

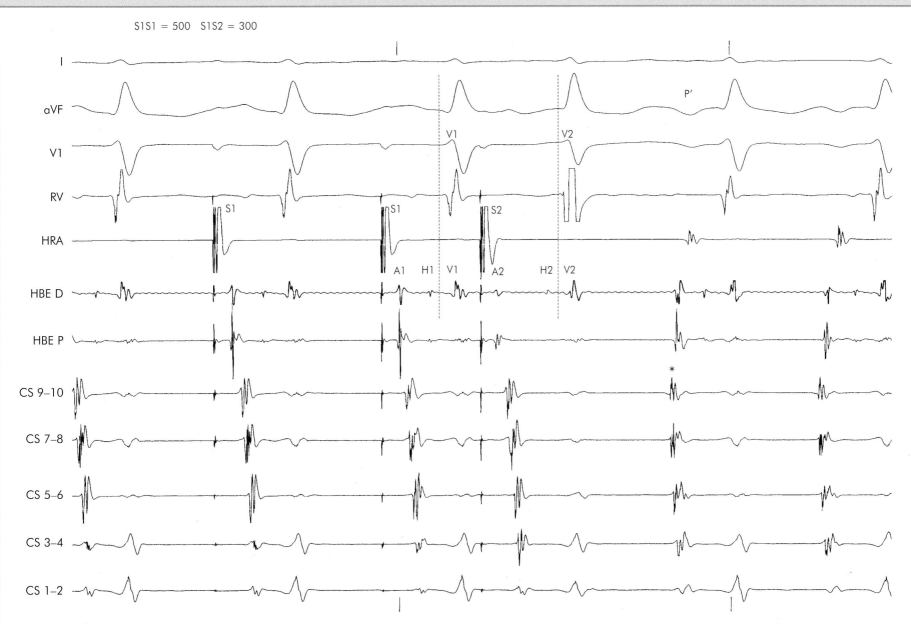

Tracing 2.3a-ii The same atrial drive train is delivered as in Tracing 2.3a-i, but the coupling interval of the extrastimulus is now shorter (S1S2 = 300 ms). Again, the SA interval and HV intervals do not change, but A2H2 has now increased to 140 ms, reflecting considerable slowing in conduction over the AV node. Note that the first spontaneous cycles after the extrastimulus do not originate in the sinus node, but around the low atrial septum, as indicated by the inverted P-wave (P') in the aVF electrogram, and the earliest atrial activation originates in the proximal coronary sinus electrogram (*). This is quite a common occurrence.

Figure 2.3a-iii illustrates that, with coupling intervals that are shorter still, the atrial extrastimuli become blocked, usually because the AV node itself is refractory (though conduction block occasionally occurs elsewhere).

2.3B ATRIAL REFRACTORINESS

If extrastimulus testing is continued with progressively shorter coupling intervals, a point is eventually reached at which the atrial tissue itself is refractory and is no longer captured (see Section 2.4B for a fuller description).

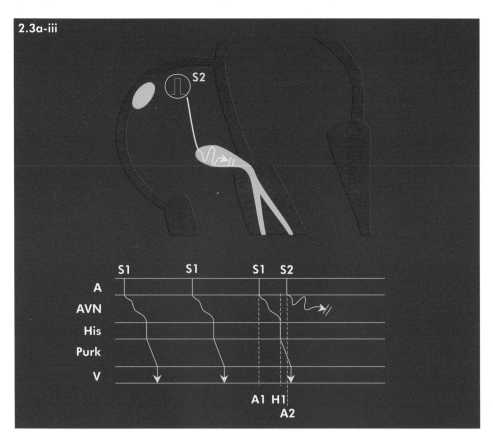

2.3a-iii

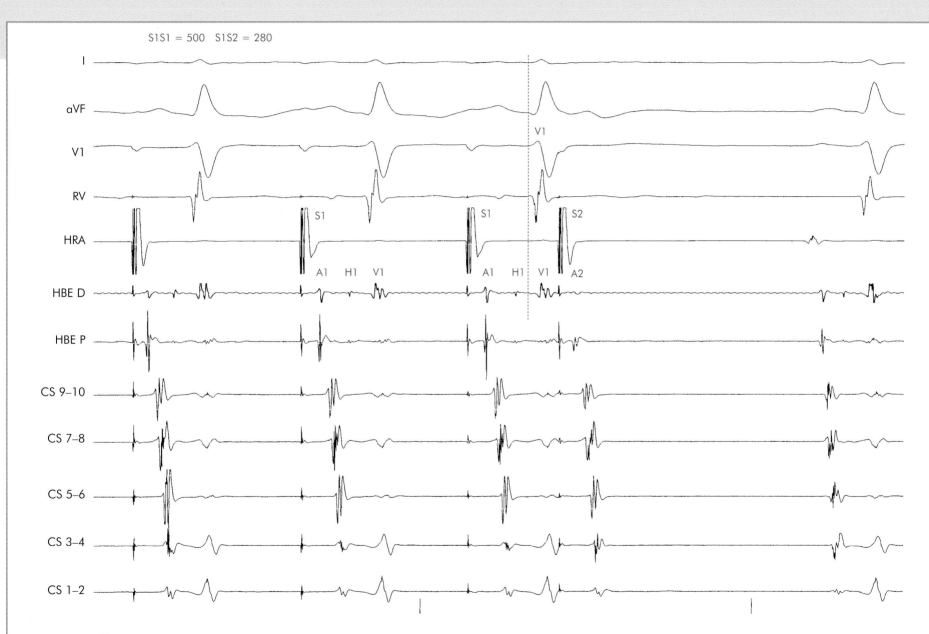

S1S1 = 500   S1S2 = 280

Tracing 2.3a-iii Further to Tracing 2.3a-ii, an extrastimulus with a slightly shorter coupling interval (280 ms) is now delivered. This is conducted to the low right atrium (LRA) without slowing (A1A2 = 280 ms) but is blocked in the AV node; in the His bundle electrogram, A2 is not followed by a His deflection and there is no subsequent ventricular depolarization.

Ventricular extrastimulus testing is carried out in a similar fashion, typically using eight-beat drive trains followed by extrastimuli with progressively shorter coupling intervals. This provides an opportunity to test retrograde conduction over the His-Purkinje system and the AV node, and to detect the presence of accessory pathways (see Section 5). Ventricular extrastimulus testing is also used for arrhythmia induction (see Sections 6 and 7). Stimulation is conventionally at the right ventricular apex, from where impulses rapidly invade the His-Purkinje system via the distal right bundle branch. If stimulation is performed at another location, activation may take longer to travel to the AV node, and allowance must be made for this in analyzing measurements.

2.4A RETROGRADE CONDUCTION OVER THE AV NODE

In a significant proportion of patients undergoing electrophysiological testing, ventriculoatrial (VA) conduction over the node can be demonstrated either at baseline or with the use of atropine and/or isoproterenol (Figure 2.4a-i). The earliest part of the atrium to be depolarized is adjacent to the AV node, so the earliest atrial activation is registered by the His bundle catheter. Activation spreads out over both atria, with the coronary sinus atrial electrograms appearing in a clear proximal → distal sequence, and the high right atrial electrogram is usually at least 30 ms after the atrial electrogram registered by the His bundle catheter. This is termed 'concentric atrial activation'.

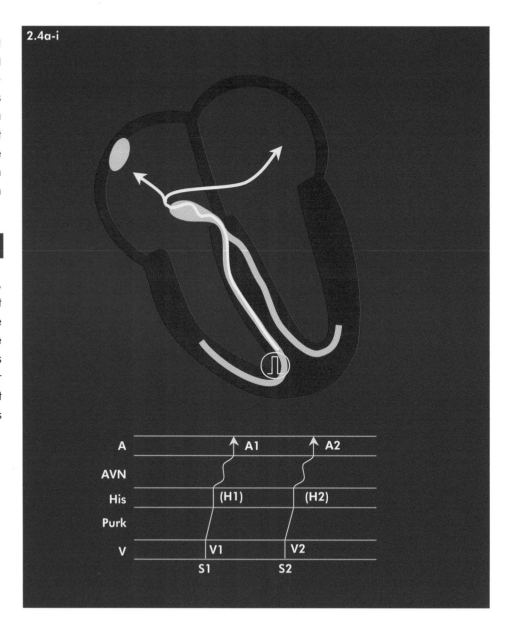

2.4a-i

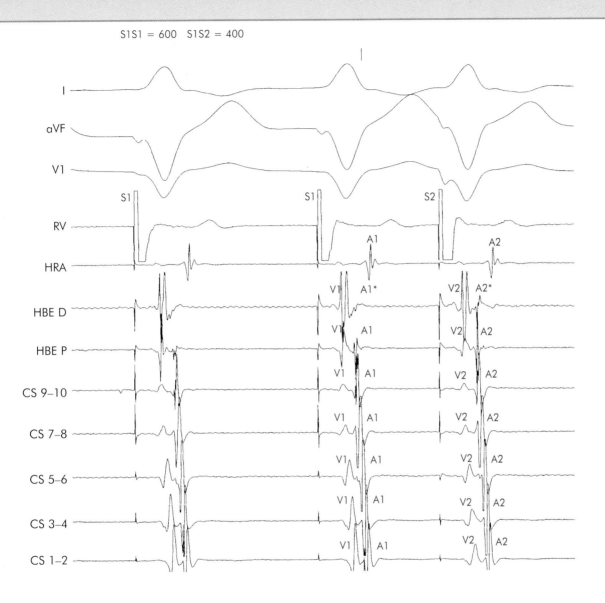

S1S1 = 600   S1S2 = 400

I

aVF

V1

RV

HRA

HBE D

HBE P

CS 9–10

CS 7–8

CS 5–6

CS 3–4

CS 1–2

Tracing 2.4a-i Extrastimulus testing at the right ventricular apex. The last two cycles of an eight-beat drive train at 600 ms cycle length (S1S1) are shown, followed by an extrastimulus (S2) with a coupling interval of 400 ms. The VA time (from earliest ventricular to earliest atrial activation) is the same for the drive train and the extrastimulus, so at this coupling interval VA conduction is non-decremental. There is a concentric pattern of atrial activation as the earliest signals (A1*, A2*) are recorded by the His bundle catheter. Note that the His bundle activation is usually not clearly seen, as it is usually buried within the ventricular signal on the His bundle electrogram. However, the His bundle deflection may become manifest if it is large relative to the ventricular deflection, or if it is late due to delay in the His-Purkinje system — quite a common finding (see Section 4.3).

With increasingly premature ventricular extrastimuli, decremental conduction in the His-Purkinje system and/or AV node begins to cause prolongation of the VA interval (Figure 2.4a-ii).

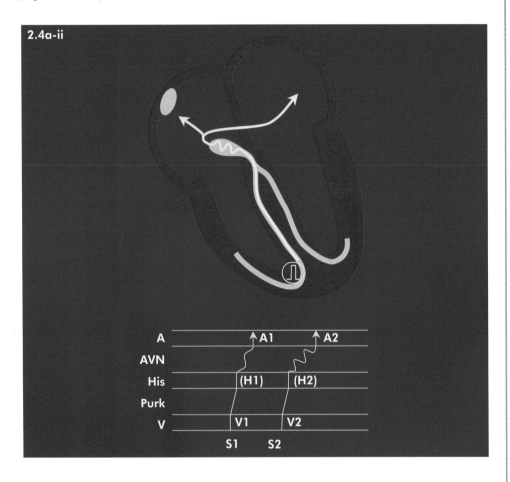

2.4a-ii

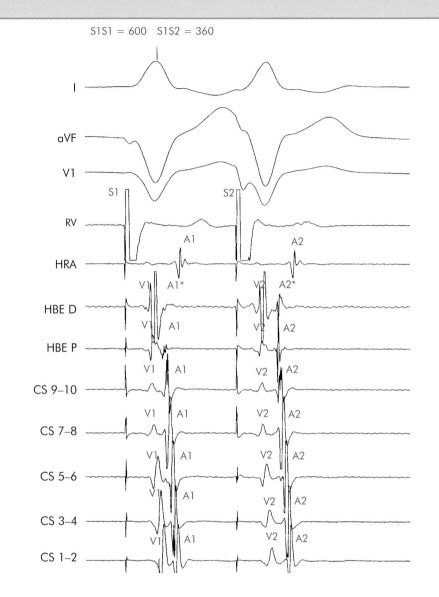

Tracing 2.4a-ii When the extrastimulus coupling interval is reduced to 360 ms, VA conduction is slightly slowed, so that V2A2 > V1A1 (onset of decremental VA conduction). However, the concentric pattern of atrial activation is unchanged.

As shown in Figure 2.4a-iii, when the ventricular extrastimuli become more premature, prolongation of the VA interval becomes pronounced, but the concentric pattern of atrial activation is unchanged.

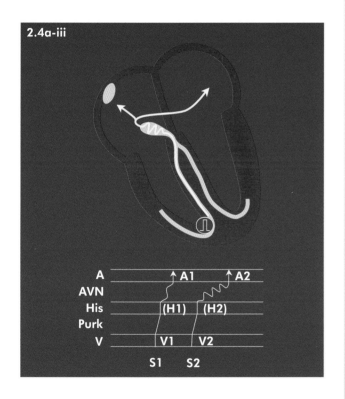

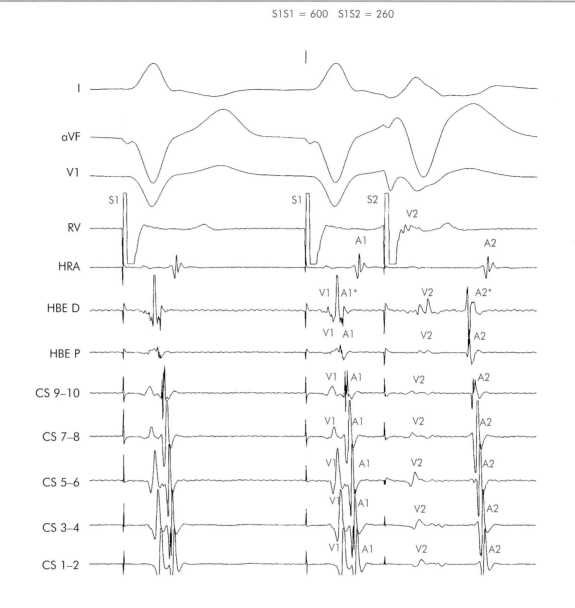

Tracing 2.4a-iii With a coupling interval of 260 ms, marked slowing in VA conduction occurs, but again the pattern of atrial activation is unchanged.

Eventually, retrograde conduction is blocked when the His-Purkinje system or AV node becomes refractory. This point is often highly dependent on the drive cycle length (Figure 2.4a-iv).

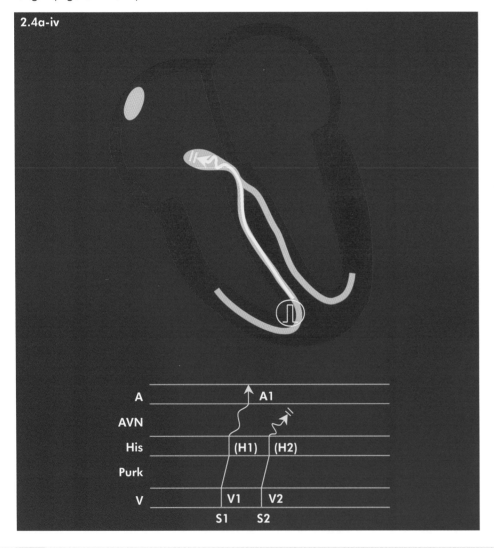

2.4a-iv

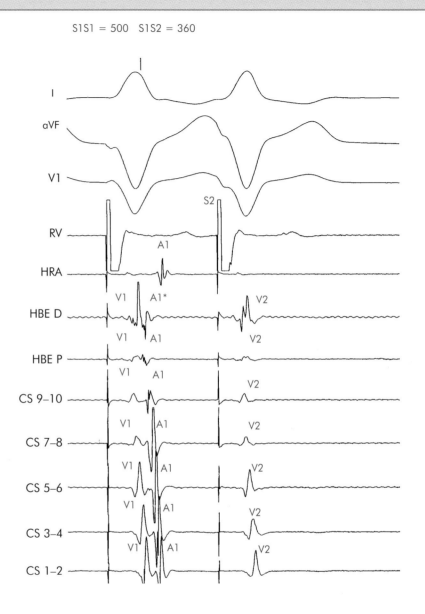

Tracing 2.4a-iv In the same patient, using a basic cycle length of 500 ms, VA block now occurs with extrastimulus coupling intervals of 360 ms and below. This illustrates the observation that the refractoriness of the retrograde conduction system can vary markedly with the basic cycle length.

It is not usually obvious to what extent decremental VA conduction is due to delay in the His-Purkinje system, and to what extent it is due to delay in the AV node. However, in some cases a retrograde His electrogram can be discerned. This usually indicates that conduction delay during ventricular extrastimulus testing is chiefly in the His-Purkinje system (i.e. VH interval prolongation). Conversely, delay in retrograde conduction during incremental ventricular pacing (Figure 2.7b) occurs chiefly in the node (i.e. HA interval prolongation).

Two other patterns of VA conduction may be considered 'normal'. Firstly, in many patients, VA conduction cannot be demonstrated at any cycle length, even with the adjunctive use of pharmacological stimuli. Secondly, it is not unusual for the retrograde exit site from the AV node to be closer to the coronary sinus ostium than the bundle of His. This results in earliest atrial activation registered in the proximal coronary sinus electrogram rather than the His bundle electrogram. However, a normal pattern of decremental conduction is still seen. If there is any doubt, a number of maneuvers are discussed in Section 5 to aid the distinction between retrograde conduction over the AV node and that over an accessory pathway.

2.4B   VENTRICULAR REFRACTORINESS

If ventricular extrastimulus testing is continued with progressively shorter coupling intervals, the ventricular refractory period is eventually reached and the ventricle is no longer captured (see Figure 2.4b). Just before this point is reached, marked delay may occur between the extrastimulus itself and the electrogram generated by the tissue. This is termed 'latency', and indicates that the extrastimulus is impinging on the refractory period of the adjacent myocardium.

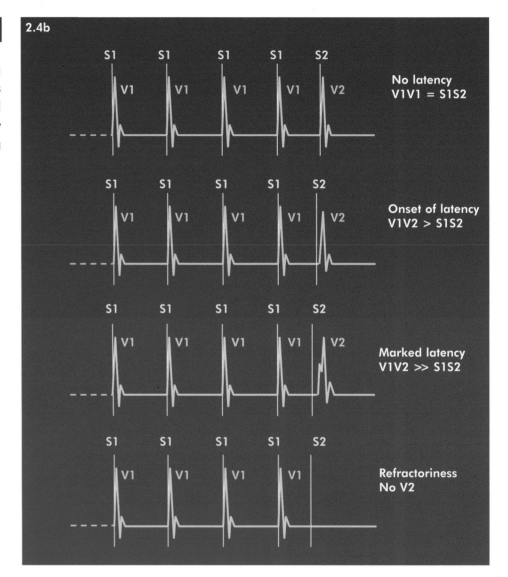

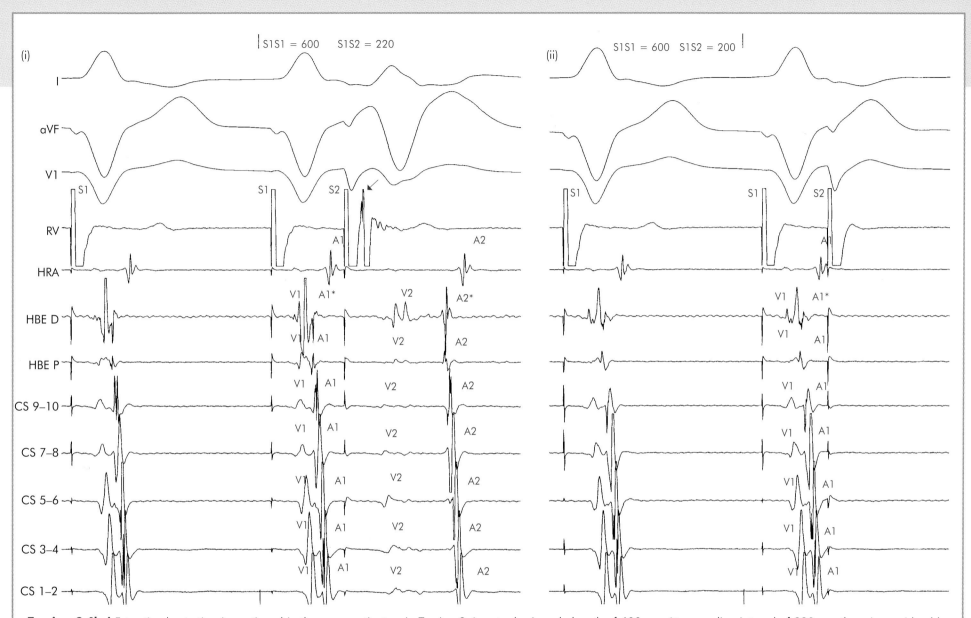

Tracing 2.4b-i Extrastimulus testing is continued in the same patient as in Tracing 2.4a, at a basic cycle length of 600 ms. At a coupling interval of 220 ms, there is considerable tissue latency, so that the local evoked response (arrowed) occurs some time after the stimulus, and V1V2 >> S1S2. A high degree of latency such as this usually occurs just above the refractory period of the tissue. As a result of this stimulus latency, the coupling interval of the impulse ascending the VA conduction system (V1V2) is at least 270 ms. This is greater than the retrograde refractory period of the VA conduction system, so the impulse is conducted back to the atria.

Tracing 2.4b-ii At a coupling interval of 200 ms, the extrastimulus no longer captures the ventricle.

2.5A EFFECTIVE, FUNCTIONAL AND RELATIVE REFRACTORY PERIODS

Refractoriness of myocardial tissue or of a conducting structure can be expressed using three measures. By far the most common measure is the 'effective refractory period', which indicates the lower limit of the input to which the tissue or structure responds.

The effective refractory period (ERP) of a tissue or structure is the longest coupling interval that fails to capture the tissue or be conducted over the structure.

Near its ERP, a structure may propagate an impulse, but with some delay (because of latency where tissue capture is being considered, and decremental conduction in a structure such as the AV node). Thus the coupling interval of the output impulse is longer than that of the input impulse.

The second most common measure of refractoriness is the 'functional refractory period', which indicates the lower limit of the output that the tissue or structure can produce.

The functional refractory period (FRP) of a tissue or structure is the shortest 'output' coupling interval that can be elicited from a tissue or structure by any 'input' interval.

The least commonly used measure of refractoriness is the 'relative refractory period', which is the point at which latency or decremental conduction begins to occur.

The relative refractory period (RRP) is the 'input' interval to a tissue or structure at which the 'output' interval just begins to differ from the 'input' interval.[†]

If extrastimulus testing shows capture without demonstrable latency right down to refractoriness, the ERP and the FRP of the tissue are identical and there is no RRP. Likewise, if a structure (such as the His-Purkinje system and most accessory pathways) is observed to conduct with no slowing until it is refractory, then again its ERP and FRP are identical and there is no RRP.

In all tissues, the ERP and FRP are cycle length-dependent and it is conventional to measure these parameters using at least two basic cycle lengths (e.g. 600 and 400 ms) for the drive train. Tracings of extrastimulus testing should therefore be annotated with the coupling intervals of both the drive cycle and the extrastimulus (e.g. S1S1 = 600 ms, S1S2 = 400 ms).

[†]Note that the RRP has a different meaning in clinical electrophysiology from that in the basic laboratory, where it refers to the interval towards the end of repolarization during which the tissue is excitable with a large stimulus but not a small one.

To take the example of antegrade conduction over the AV node:

The AV node ERP (AVNERP) is the longest A1A2 interval (measured from the His bundle electrogram[††]) that fails to be conducted to the His bundle.

The AV node FRP (AVNFRP) is the shortest H1H2 interval that can be elicited by any A1A2 interval.

Again, it is correct to measure H1H2 as the direct output of the AV node, and not V1V2. The latter measurement may give an erroneous result if there is variation in the HV interval (though this is unusual).

The AV node RRP (AVNRRP) is the longest A1A2 interval at which A2H2 exceeds A1H1 (or H1H2 exceeds A1A2).

In the patient illustrated in Tracing 2.3a, at a basic cycle length of 500 ms, the AVNERP was 280 ms, the AVNFRP was 340 ms and the AVNRRP was 440 ms.

To take another example, the following are the refractory measures relating to capture of the ventricular myocardium:

The ventricular ERP (VERP) is the longest S1S2 interval that fails to capture the myocardium.

The ventricular FRP (VFRP) is the shortest V1V2 that can be elicited by any S1S2 interval.

The ventricular RRP (VRRP) is the longest S1S2 interval at which S2V2 exceeds S1V1 (or V1V2 exceeds S1S2).

In the patient illustrated in Tracing 2.4b, at a basic cycle length of 600 ms, the VERP was 200 ms, the VFRP was 270 ms and the VRRP was 280 ms.

Normal values for refractory periods are listed on page 238.

[††]This is very important as it is the best estimate of the 'input' coupling interval to the AV node. Due to latency in atrial capture and intra-atrial conduction delay, A1A2 may be significantly greater than the extrastimulus coupling interval S1S2.

2.5B THE ANTEGRADE CONDUCTION CURVE

Figure 2.5b illustrates conduction over the AV node during atrial extrastimulus testing. A1A2 measured from the His bundle catheter is plotted on the abscissa. H1H2 (the coupling interval with which the extrastimulus is propagated out of the AV node) and A2H2 (the conduction time of the extrastimulus over the AV node) are plotted on the ordinate. The red dashed line is the line of identity between the axes.

Note that for A1A2 intervals of 380 ms and greater, A2H2 is constant and H1H2 = A1A2, keeping to the line of identity. Over this part of the curve, conduction is non-decremental. As A1A2 intervals decrease below 380 ms, there is progressive slowing in conduction of the extrastimulus, whereby A2H2 increases and H1H2 progressively departs from the line of identity. Conduction is decremental over this part of the curve, which has a typical 'hockey-stick' shape. The shortest A1A2 interval to be conducted is 290 ms: intervals of 280 ms and lower are not conducted. The AVNERP is therefore estimated at 280 ms. The shortest H1H2 achieved is 370 ms, which is the AVNFRP. The AVNRRP is 380 ms, the start of the decremental part of the curve.

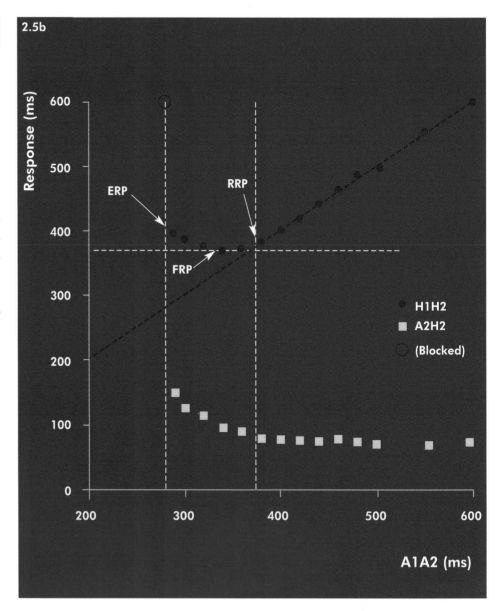

Determination of refractory periods using 10 ms or even 20 ms steps in the extrastimulus coupling interval is sufficient for most clinical purposes. Smaller steps can be used if greater accuracy is required, e.g. for a research protocol. In certain circumstances, however, it can be difficult to determine refractory periods and some examples are outlined below.

Accurate estimation of retrograde AV node ERP

The 'input' to the AV node during ventricular stimulation is through the bundle of His, so by definition the retrograde AVNERP is the longest H1H2 interval that fails to be conducted over the node back up to the atria. In practice, however, the retrograde His potential is usually buried within the ventricular electrogram registered by the His catheter, and cannot be measured. In this situation, it is preferable to refer to the retrograde ERP of the VA conduction system, rather than that of the node. Likewise, it can be difficult to determine the onset of the ventricular electrogram after the stimulus artifact, and S1S2 may have to be used as a surrogate for V1V2.

In the example illustrated in Tracing 2.4, the exact onset of ventricular activation is not clear from the surface or intracardiac signals, though it is clear by 2.4a (iii) and 2.4b (i) that V2 has become widely separated from S2. No retrograde His is clearly seen at any point.

AV node conduction down to tissue refractoriness

As atrial extrastimulus coupling intervals are progressively reduced, it is not uncommon for the AV node to continue to conduct right down to the point at which the extrastimulus fails to capture the atrium. This may be because the AV nodal ERP is less than the atrial ERP, or because there is sufficient delay in the atrium that the coupling interval of the impulse arriving at the node remains above the AVNERP. In this situation, one can only state that the AVNERP is less than the shortest A1A2 that was seen, and the AVNFRP is less than or equal to the shortest H1H2 seen. The same problem frequently occurs with measurements of retrograde conduction.

Again, in the example illustrated in Tracing 2.4, retrograde conduction over the AV node continued as the extrastimulus coupling interval was decreased, until S1S2 = 200 ms, when the ventricular tissue was no longer captured. The shortest V1V2 measured (VFRP) was 270 ms, so it can be stated that the retrograde ERP of the VA conduction system is <270 ms.

The 'gap' phenomenon

Conduction of an impulse may be blocked at a certain S1S2 interval, then reappear as the S1S2 interval is lowered, only to disappear finally at a lower level still. The mechanism of this discontinuity in conduction is usually apparent, and caused by a 'gap' phenomenon, described in Section 2.6A. In this situation, conduction is conventionally assumed to have ceased when block first disappears (i.e. the highest S1S2 that results in a non-conducted impulse), and measurements are related to this point.

Arrhythmia induction

Extrastimulus testing around the AVNERP may be hampered by the repeated induction of supraventricular tachycardias (see Sections 4–6). The risk of inducing sustained atrial or ventricular arrhythmias increases as the extrastimulus coupling interval falls. The clinician must balance the wish to obtain a complete study against the potential inconvenience and even risk of arrhythmia induction. Some centers do not routinely use extrastimuli with coupling intervals <200 ms, or will discontinue extrastimulus testing at the point at which frequent atrial or ventricular repetitive responses are seen.

As the coupling interval of an extrastimulus is progressively decreased, propagation of the resulting impulse is sometimes seen to cease at one point, then resume at a shorter extrastimulus coupling interval.

2.6A   GAP PHENOMENON

The gap phenomenon is by far the most common explanation of apparent paradoxical conduction. It can occur when an impulse is conducted over two structures in sequence, with the first having a shorter ERP than the second, e.g. the AV node and the His-Purkinje system (with conduction over the latter affected by gap physiology). Because of delay in the proximal structure, a decrease in the coupling interval of an extrastimulus may result in the propagated impulse arriving at the second structure with an increased coupling interval.

In Figure 2.6a-i, an extrastimulus is conducted with left bundle branch block, because H1H2 is less than the ERP of the left bundle branch (LBB ERP). In Figure 2.6a-ii, a slightly earlier extrastimulus is conducted with greater decrement over the AV node. Now the resulting H1H2 is greater than the LBB ERP, so conduction to the ventricles is normal.

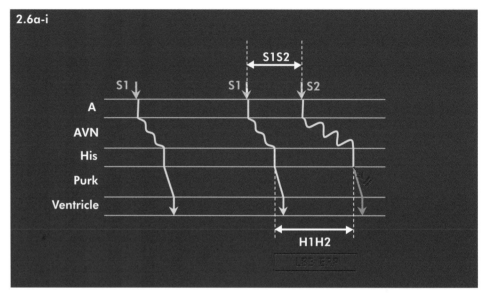

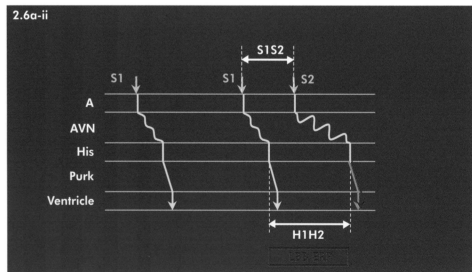

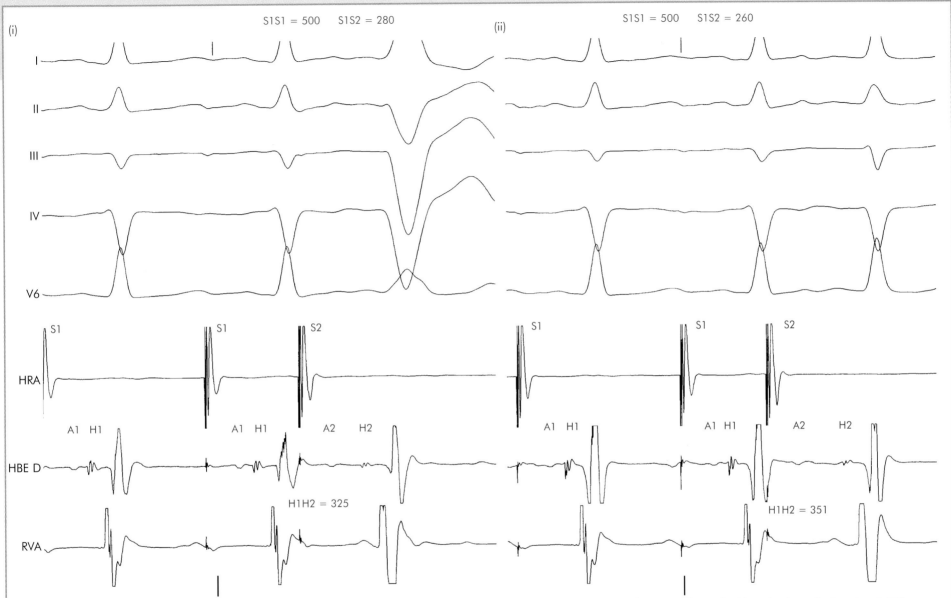

Tracing 2.6a Gap phenomenon affecting conduction over the left bundle branch. Atrial extrastimulus testing is being performed with a basic cycle length of 500 ms. 2.6a-i With an extrastimulus coupling interval of 280 ms, the impulse is conducted normally over the AV node, but there is a left bundle branch block in the His-Purkinje system. 2.6a-ii When the extrastimulus coupling interval is reduced to 260 ms, the impulse is conducted without bundle branch block.

The explanation for the apparently paradoxical return of conduction in the left bundle branch is provided by examination of the A2H2 and H1H2 intervals; these coupling intervals are on the steeply decremental portion of the AV nodal conduction curve, during which the AH interval rises markedly. Consequently, as S1S2 is reduced by 20 ms, H1H2 increases by 26 ms and this brings H1H2 outside the LBB ERP, so aberrant conduction disappears. This mechanism is illustrated in Figures 2.6a (i)-(ii).

Gap physiology may also affect conduction through the atrial myocardium and over the AV node. In Figure 2.6a-iii, an extrastimulus (S2) delivered in the high right atrium arrives at the AV node (A2) when it is refractory (A1A2 < AVNERP), and conduction is therefore blocked. In Figure 2.6a-iv, an earlier extrastimulus is delayed by latency and slowed conduction in the atrium. The propagated impulse now arrives at the AV node when the latter is no longer refractory (A1A2 > AVNERP), and is therefore conducted.

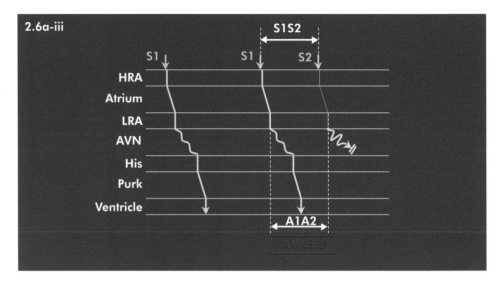

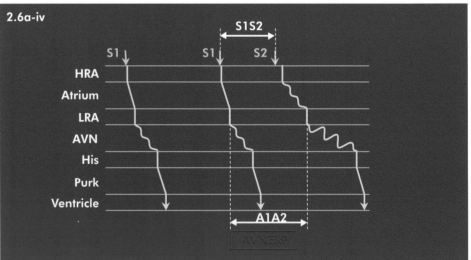

2.6B   OTHER MECHANISMS OF 'PARADOXICAL' CONDUCTION

Conduction over a structure may occur unexpectedly for other reasons. For example: a change in preceding cycle length, causing shortening of refractoriness, is an extremely common explanation (illustrated in Tracings 2.4a). 'Peeling back refractoriness' is a mechanism whereby self-sustained bundle branch block during tachycardia may be terminated by a premature ventricular complex (for an example, see Tracing 6.5b). True 'supernormal conduction' is a phenomenon described in the basic laboratory, but very difficult to prove in clinical practice: during tissue repolarization (phase III), a brief window may exist during which tissue excitability and conduction are improved.

In addition to extrastimulus testing, other pacing protocols, especially incremental pacing, are routinely used during diagnostic electrophysiologic testing.

2.7A INCREMENTAL ATRIAL PACING

The other stimulation protocol in routine use for diagnostic EP study is incremental pacing. Atrial incremental pacing involves stimulation (usually by the high right atrial catheter) at a constant cycle length slightly shorter than that of the patient's spontaneous rhythm. The pacing cycle length is then decreased in small steps while the rhythm is observed for several seconds between each step. In contrast to extrastimulus testing, the purpose of this mode of stimulation is to observe impulse propagation during steady-state conditions. The principal observation is the cycle length at which 1:1 conduction over the AV node ceases. This is widely known as the Wenckebach cycle length (WCL) and is illustrated in Figure 2.7a.

A number of other observations may be made during incremental pacing, including: a sudden increase in the AH interval (suggesting dual AV nodal physiology; see Section 4); ventricular pre-excitation via an accessory pathway (see Section 5); or arrhythmia induction (see Sections 3–6).

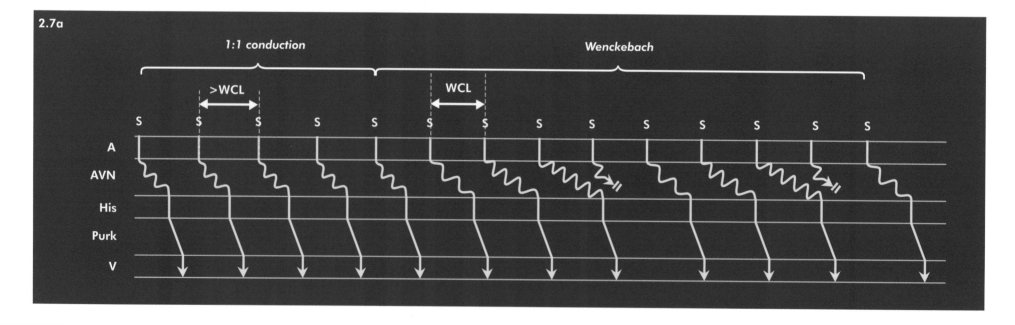

2.7a

1:1 conduction   Wenckebach

>WCL   WCL

S S S S S S S S S S S S S S S

A

AVN

His

Purk

V

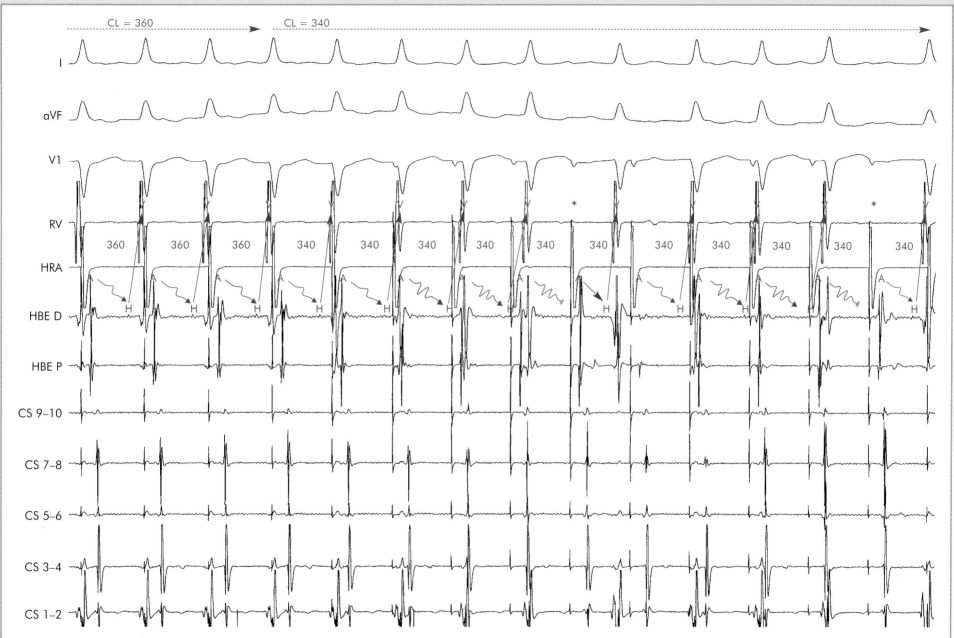

Tracing 2.7a Incremental atrial pacing. The first three cycles show the end of a sequence of pacing at 360 ms in the high right atrium. At this cycle length, there is considerable slowing in conduction over the AV node, resulting in an AH interval of ≈200 ms. When the pacing cycle length is reduced to 340 ms, Wenckebach-type atrioventricular block occurs with a progressive increase in AH interval, resulting eventually in a blocked cycle (*). The atrioventricular Wenckebach cycle length (AV WCL) is 340 ms.

2.7B   INCREMENTAL VENTRICULAR PACING

Incremental ventricular pacing follows the same principles as incremental atrial pacing (Figure 2.7b). The principal interests are the cycle length at which 1:1 VA conduction ceases (although, the mode of VA block in VA WCL may not actually be a typical 'Wenckebach' pattern) and the pattern and timing of retrograde atrial activation (see Sections 4 and 5).

2.7C   OTHER PROTOCOLS

Multiple extrastimuli may be used for arrhythmia induction (e.g. programmed ventricular stimulation; see Section 7). 'Long-short' stimulus sequences may be needed to provoke certain arrhythmias or patterns of conduction block (e.g. in bundle branches where this is of interest).

A 'step-up' protocol may be used to estimate the ERP of a tissue; i.e. the initial extrastimulus coupling interval is very short (e.g. 100 ms) and this is progressively increased until tissue capture is achieved. This avoids repeated extrastimuli just above the ERP, and may reduce the risk of arrhythmia induction.

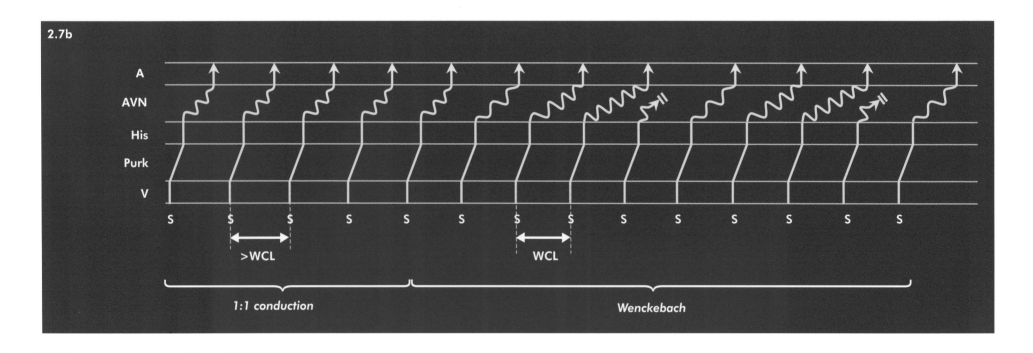

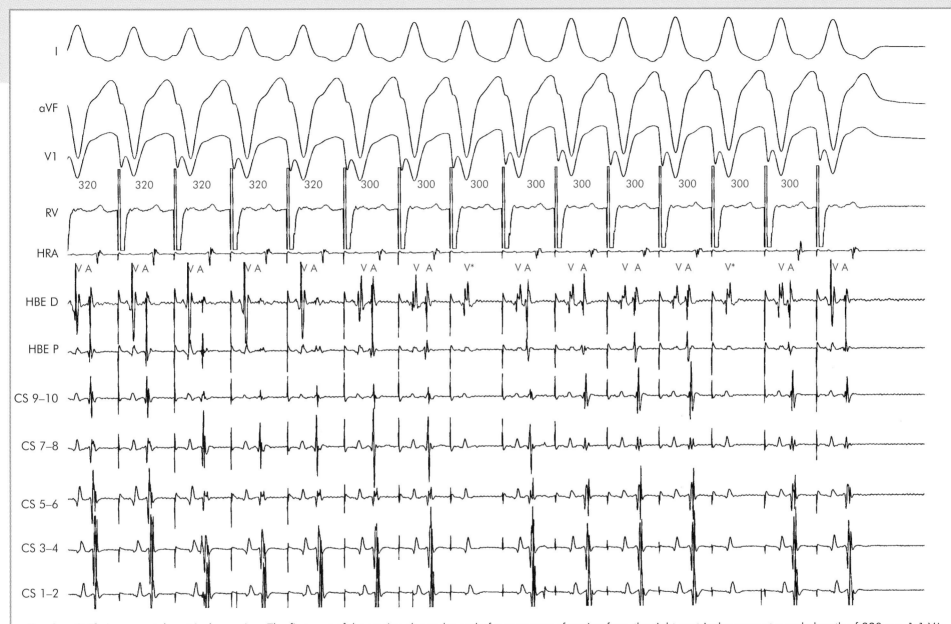

Tracing 2.7b Incremental ventricular pacing. The first part of the tracing shows the end of a sequence of pacing from the right ventricular apex at a cycle length of 320 ms. 1:1 VA conduction is seen. When the ventricular cycle length is reduced to 300 ms, intermittent VA block is seen (*). The VA WCL is recorded as 300 ms, though VA block does not follow a classical Wenckebach pattern of VA prolongation prior to block; it is possible that the block is occurring in the His-Purkinje system below the AV node.

All EP laboratories have developed their own protocols over time. The following is one suggestion for a minimum protocol of testing. Further electrophysiologic exploration, as described in the following chapters, can be individualized according to the findings at this baseline study and the clinical information available.

- **Measurement of basic intervals**

  This establishes whether a long PR interval is due to slow conduction in the AV node or the His-Purkinje system (or both), and may indicate whether a short PR interval is due to ventricular pre-excitation (see Section 5).

  Measurements: rhythm, cycle length, PA, AH, HV, QRS, QRS morphology if abnormal, QT and QTc

- **Assessment of SNRT at basic cycle lengths (BCLs) of 800, 600, 500, 400 and 350 ms**

  An abnormal SNRT may indicate sinus node dysfunction as a cause for symptoms (see Section 2.2A).

  Measurement: maximum CSNRT

- **Ventricular extrastimulus testing down to ventricular refractoriness at basic cycle lengths of 600 and 400 ms**

  This indicates the presence or absence of retrograde conduction, and allows measurement of the ERP and FRP of the VA conduction system, and of the ERP and FRP of ventricular myocardium (see Sections 2.4 and 2.5). A basic cycle length of 700 ms or longer may be necessary if VA conduction is otherwise absent, and a shorter basic cycle length may be necessary in a patient with marked resting sinus tachycardia.

  Eccentric retrograde atrial activation or VA conduction that is non-decremental or shows discontinuity may indicate the presence of an accessory AV pathway (see Section 5) or dual AV nodal physiology (see Section 4). Ventricular tachycardia (VT) may be induced by a single extrastimulus (see Section 7).

  Measurements: VERP and retrograde AVNERP at both cycle lengths

- **Incremental ventricular pacing from slightly faster than sinus rhythm down to VA Wenckebach point, or a minimum cycle length of 300 ms**

  If VA conduction is present, VA WCL can be measured. Pacing is usually not faster than a cycle length of 300 ms, and may stop at a slower rate if it is poorly tolerated.

  Measurement: VA WCL

- **Atrial extrastimulus testing down to refractoriness at cycle lengths of 600 and 400 ms**

  This allows the measurement of AV nodal ERP and FRP, and atrial ERP and FRP (see Sections 2.3 and 2.5); longer or shorter basic cycle lengths may be needed in certain circumstances.

  Dual AV nodal physiology (see Section 4) or ventricular pre-excitation (see Section 5) may be demonstrated and atrial arrhythmias may also be induced (see Section 3).

  Measurements: AVNERP, AVNFRP and AERP at both cycle lengths

- **Incremental atrial pacing from slightly faster than sinus rhythm down to AV Wenckebach point, or a minimum cycle length of 300 ms**

  This will permit measurement of AV Wenckebach cycle length and thus establish whether rate-dependent AV block occurs in the node (AH block) or below (HV block) (see Section 2.7A). Again, pacing is usually not faster than a cycle length of 300 ms during basic testing, and may stop at a slower rate if poorly tolerated.

  Measurement: AV WCL

The minimum protocol evolved largely for the diagnosis of supraventricular tachycardias (SVTs). However, the protocol is seldom sufficient to achieve a 'complete' positive diagnosis, or completely to exclude an arrhythmic cause for symptoms. Atrial stimulation is more likely than ventricular stimulation to induce SVTs, such as atrial tachycardia and AV nodal reentry, and incremental atrial pacing in particular carries a risk of causing atrial fibrillation. It is therefore our habit to perform ventricular stimulation studies first in patients with suspected SVTs or atrial arrhythmias. This order also has the advantage that, if VA conduction is completely absent, AV reentry (see Section 5) and AV nodal reentrant tachycardia (AVNRT; see Section 4) are very unlikely and can often be ruled out at an early stage. For the same reason, in a patient with a suspected diagnosis of ventricular tachycardia, it is reasonable to commence with atrial studies.

Depending on the clinical background to the study, and the findings from baseline testing, a number of other maneuvers can be added.

Suspected sinus node disease

• More detailed node testing of sinus node function (measurement of SACT — see Section 2).

Suspected ventricular tachycardia

• Programmed ventricular stimulation using multiple extrastimuli (see Section 7). Short-long-short induction sequences may facilitate induction of bundle branch reentry.

Suspected AV nodal reentry or atrial arrhythmias

• Intravenous isoproterenol and/or atropine. These can also be administered if VA conduction is absent or poor at baseline.

• Atrial extrastimulus testing at different cycle lengths, using double, triple or more atrial extrastimuli.

The above maneuvers are particularly helpful in the situation, frequently encountered, where dual AV nodal physiology has been encountered, but AV nodal reentrant tachycardia has not yet been induced (see Section 4).

Suspected accessory AV pathway

• Pacing at sites other than the high right atrium and right ventricular apex may demonstrate the presence of accessory pathways (see Section 5). Again, intravenous isoproterenol and/or atropine may facilitate tachycardia induction, usually by improving conduction over the AV node.

Pacing and drug administration during tachycardia

The differential diagnosis of narrow- and wide-complex tachycardia is discussed in detail in Sections 6 and 7, and is summarized at the end of Section 9.

FURTHER READING

1. Josephson ME. Clinical Cardiac Electrophysiology. Second edition. Philadelphia/London: Lea and Febiger, 1993:12–166.

2. Techniques in electrophysiologic testing. In: Prystowsky EN, Klein GJ. Cardiac Arrhythmias: An Integrated Approach for the Clinician. New York: McGraw-Hill, 1994:299–334.

3. Reiffel JA, Kuehnert MJ. Electrophysiological testing of sinus node function: diagnostic and prognostic application-including updated information from sinus node electrograms. Pacing Clin Electrophysiol 1994;17(3 Pt 1):349–65.

4. Yee R, Strauss HC. Electrophysiologic mechanisms: sinus node dysfunction. Circulation 1987;75(4 Pt 2):III12–8.

5. Wu D, Denes P, Dhingra R et al. Nature of the gap phenomenon in man. Circ Res 1974;34(5):682–92.

6. Childers RW. Supernormality. Cardiovasc Clin 1973;5(3):135–58.

The terminology used to describe arrhythmias is a source of constant confusion. We shall use the term 'atrial' to describe those arrhythmias in which the entire substrate is within the atria and does not involve the atrioventricular (AV) node. To confirm the diagnosis of an atrial arrhythmia in the electrophysiology (EP) laboratory, it is necessary to demonstrate that the arrhythmia can continue without the participation of the AV node.

Even among the atrial arrhythmias, there are differences with respect to nomenclature. It is conventional to differentiate between atrial tachycardia and atrial flutter according to the P-wave cycle length on the surface ECG. Thus, an atrial arrhythmia with a cycle length between ~250–500 ms (rate between 120–240 beats/min) is conventionally referred to as 'atrial tachycardia'. If the cycle length is shorter (<220 ms, rate >270 beats/min), the arrhythmia is termed 'atrial flutter'. This convention has the advantage of allowing a label to be given to an arrhythmia at the bedside. Unfortunately, the convention does not always correspond with the arrhythmia mechanism (for example, the use of antiarrhythmic drugs in a patient with typical atrial flutter may increase the cycle length to >250 ms, though the arrhythmia mechanism remains the same).

This section will discuss methods for determining the source and mechanism of atrial arrhythmias, and a more mechanistic classification will therefore be used. For the purpose of this discussion, we have divided the atrial arrhythmias into four groups: (i) those arising from the region of the sinus node; (ii) those arising from a circumscribed 'focus' (a source of enhanced automaticity or triggered activity, or a micro-reentrant circuit) elsewhere in the atria, which we shall call 'atrial tachycardia'; (iii) macro-reentrant circuits, all of which have been included under the term 'atrial flutter'; and (iv) atrial fibrillation. This classification may have shortcomings from the basic science viewpoint and is not always possible using the surface ECG, but it fits with the diagnostic and therapeutic strategies available to the clinical electrophysiologist.

Finally, we recognize that in many countries the term 'supraventricular tachycardia (SVT)' is used exclusively to refer to arrhythmias dependent on the AV junction (AV and AV nodal reentry). However, we shall follow the more widespread convention that an 'SVT' is any arrhythmia that is not ventricular — we therefore include atrial arrhythmias. The term 'SVT' will be used infrequently, and the misleading term 'paroxysmal atrial tachycardia' will be avoided altogether.

3.1 SINUS NODE TACHYCARDIAS

3.2 ATRIAL ECTOPY AND TACHYCARDIA

3.3 TYPICAL ATRIAL FLUTTER

3.4 ARRHYTHMIA ENTRAINMENT

3.5 ATYPICAL ATRIAL FLUTTERS

3.6 ATRIAL FIBRILLATION

Arrhythmias arising from the region of the sinus node are indistinguishable from physiological sinus tachycardia on the basis of the P-wave morphology and the sequence of atrial activation on intracardiac recordings. Only by examining the behavior of these rhythms can we differentiate between them.

3.1A PHYSIOLOGICAL SINUS TACHYCARDIA

Physiological sinus tachycardia is far more commonly seen (even in the EP laboratory) than any pathological arrhythmia arising from the sinus node and adjacent atrium. It is not paroxysmal, i.e. its onset and termination are gradual. The rate is sensitive to autonomic modulations, such as those associated with hypovolemia, hypoxia, pain and anxiety, and to a variety of drugs. Physiological sinus tachycardia is not initiated by pacing methods and can be suppressed, but not terminated, by overdrive pacing.

3.1B INAPPROPRIATE SINUS TACHYCARDIA

Inappropriate sinus tachycardia (also known as chronic sinus tachycardia) is a poorly understood condition. It is indistinguishable from physiological sinus tachycardia except that the increased rate (>100 beats/min) is continuous and has no apparent cause. Young women are most commonly affected. A different form of inappropriate sinus tachycardia is an exaggerated response to exercise or stress (for example, a heart rate that is normal at rest but rapidly rises to 140 beats/min on climbing stairs, in an otherwise well person). Treatment of inappropriate sinus tachycardia (if indicated at all) is generally limited to beta-blockers, although catheter modification of the sinus node is occasionally performed for patients with intractable and drug-refractory symptoms.

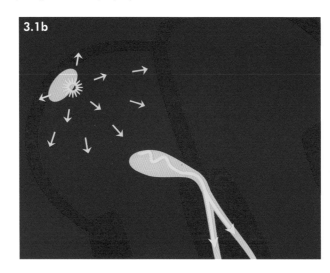

3.1C SINUS NODE REENTRY

Sinus node reentry is a distinct entity from physiological sinus tachycardia. It is a paroxysmal arrhythmia with abrupt onset and termination. At electrophysiological study, the arrhythmia can be initiated and terminated with atrial extrastimuli and the earliest atrial activation is in the sinus node region. This arrhythmia is frequently an incidental finding in the EP laboratory, rather than the cause of symptoms. When it is a clinical problem it is generally treated with antiarrhythmic drugs.

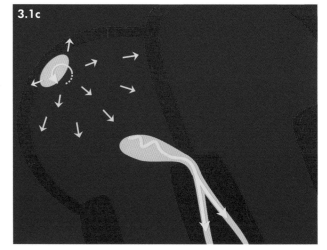

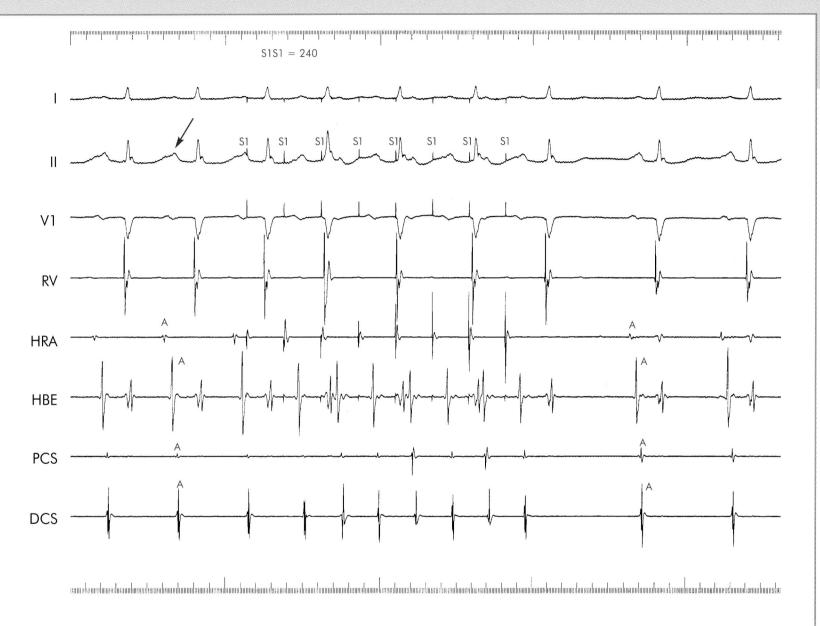

Tracing 3.1 Burst atrial pacing into a right atrial tachycardia (cycle length 450 ms), consistent with sinus node reentry. Pacing terminated the tachycardia with resumption of sinus rhythm (cycle length 600 ms). Note that the morphology of the P-wave (arrow) and the atrial activation sequence (A-A-A-A) are identical in tachycardia and in subsequent sinus rhythm. This, and the consistent induction and termination with atrial extrastimuli, makes sinus node reentry the most likely diagnosis.

Clues to the site of origin of premature atrial ectopic beats and tachycardia can be obtained from the resulting P-wave morphology. However, intracardiac recordings, even with the standard four-catheter configuration, can give a more precise location.

If the earliest activation is recorded by the His electrode, then an origin in the anteroseptal right atrium is suggested, while early activation in the proximal coronary sinus suggests a posteroseptal origin. If high and low right atrial electrograms are equally early, then an origin elsewhere in the right atrium is suggested. Similarly, a lateral left atrial focus is usually manifest earliest in the distal coronary sinus, while activation from a high left atrial focus may reach all the coronary sinus electrodes virtually simultaneously. An origin near the right superior pulmonary vein may actually reach the high right atrial electrode before the coronary sinus. Caution must therefore be exercised in interpreting recordings from static electrodes; mapping (see Section 8) is necessary to pin-point an ectopic focus with confidence.

Ectopic atrial tachycardias are regular arrhythmias arising from regions of the atria other than the sinus node. They arise from a small area of tissue but can be caused by a number of mechanisms.

3.2A MICRO-REENTRY

Micro-reentry is suggested when the arrhythmia can be consistently initiated and terminated by extrastimuli, or can be entrained (see Section 3.5).

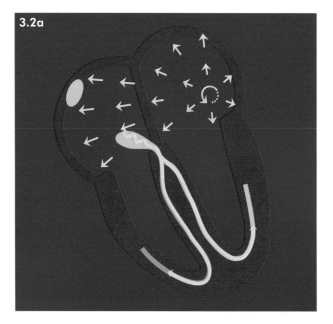

3.2a

3.2B FOCAL ATRIAL TACHYCARDIA

Truly focal (as opposed to micro-reentrant) atrial tachycardia may be the result of triggered activity or abnormal automaticity. Triggered activity is suggested when the arrhythmia is inducible by rapid pacing but there is no other evidence of reentry (such as entrainment, see Section 3.4). Abnormal automaticity is suggested when the arrhythmia cannot be induced or terminated by pacing. Pharmacological measures, such as isoproterenol infusion, are often needed to induce automatic arrhythmias in the electrophysiology laboratory.

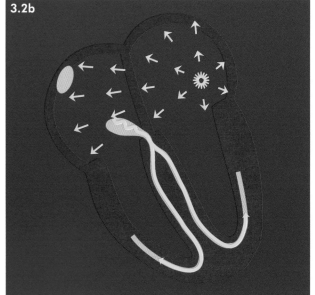

3.2b

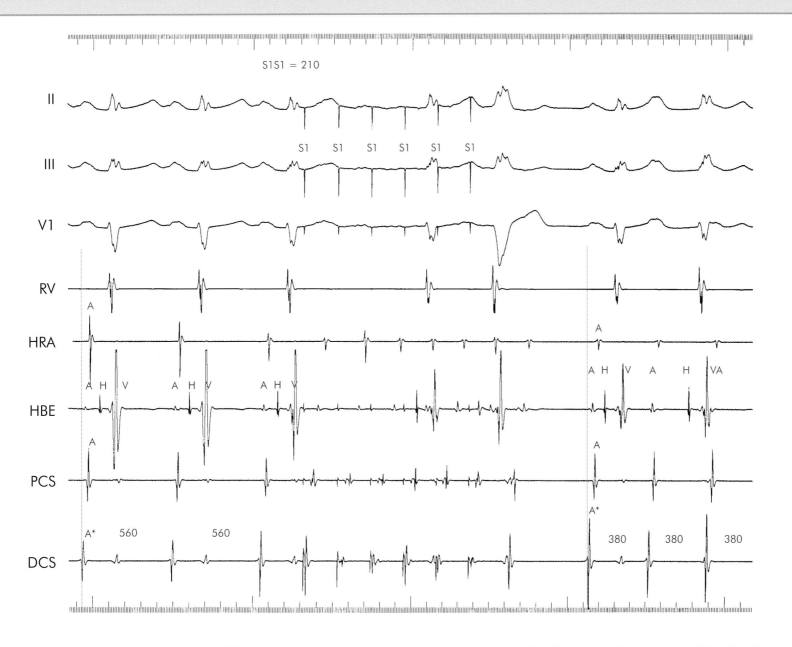

Tracing 3.2 Left atrial tachycardia (cycle length 560 ms) with earliest activation in the distal coronary sinus (A*). After a burst of atrial pacing (S1) in the distal coronary sinus (DCS), a more rapid tachycardia (cycle length 380 ms) with Wenckebach AV block is seen. The atrial activation sequence and P-wave morphology are unaltered. This is probably the same tachycardia, accelerated by the rapid pacing, indicating that triggered activity may be the mechanism.

3.3A MACRO-REENTRANT RIGHT ATRIAL CIRCUIT

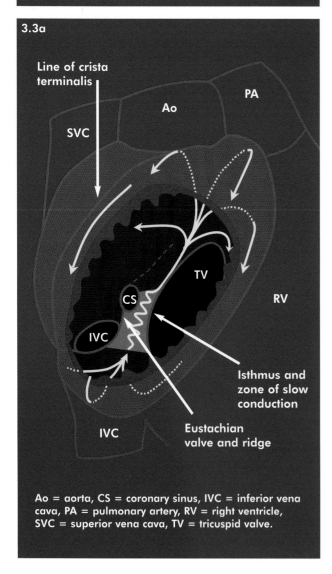

3.3a

Line of crista terminalis

PA

Ao

SVC

TV

CS

RV

IVC

IVC

Isthmus and zone of slow conduction

Eustachian valve and ridge

Ao = aorta, CS = coronary sinus, IVC = inferior vena cava, PA = pulmonary artery, RV = right ventricle, SVC = superior vena cava, TV = tricuspid valve.

Multi-electrode recordings have demonstrated that typical atrial flutter (also known as 'common' flutter) is a macro-reentrant circuit confined to the right atrium. Left atrial activation is entirely passive. Figure 3.3a depicts the right atrium, viewed from above and to the right (equivalent to a cranial right anterior oblique projection), with its anterior wall opened. The wavefront emerges from a zone of slow conduction between the tricuspid annulus and coronary sinus (CS) os, and ascends the interatrial septum, spreading to depolarize the posterior right atrium. It then crosses the roof of the right atrium and travels downward and laterally between the tricuspid valve and the crista terminalis. These structures funnel the wavefront into a narrow channel (the isthmus) between the tricuspid annulus and inferior vena cava, then back to the zone of slow conduction. A line of functional block exists along the crista terminalis where the ascending and descending wavefronts collide.

3.3B RECORDING ATRIAL FLUTTER ACTIVATION

Figure 3.3b illustrates a catheter configuration commonly used to record activation in atrial flutter, as if viewed from the apex of the heart, through the tricuspid valve (equivalent to a caudal left anterior oblique projection). A multi-electrode catheter is positioned in the right atrium with its tip in the tricuspid-IVC isthmus (shaded), and proximal poles just anterior to the crista terminalis. Other catheters are in the conventional His and CS locations.

The arrow depicts the direction of atrial activation in typical atrial flutter. The wavefront emerges from the isthmus, and the earliest signal is recorded by either the proximal CS pole or the His catheter. As activation proceeds down the lateral wall of the right atrium back to the isthmus, it is recorded in sequence by the proximal to distal poles of the multipolar catheter. CS activation is from proximal to distal.

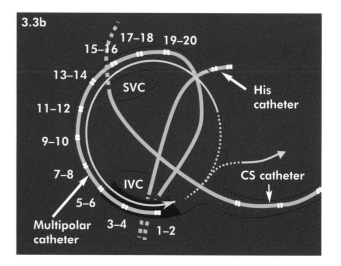

3.3b

17–18 19–20
15–16
13–14
SVC
11–12
His catheter
9–10
7–8
IVC
CS catheter
5–6
Multipolar catheter
3–4 1–2

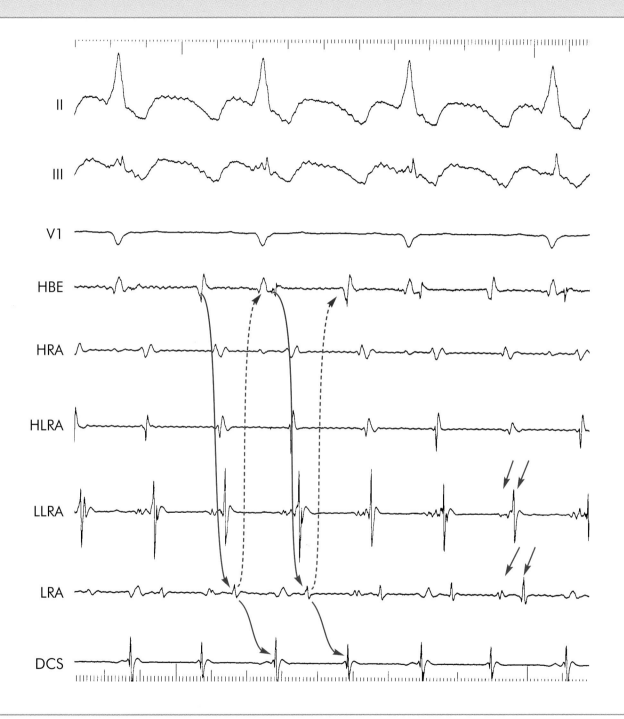

Tracing 3.3 Typical atrial flutter. On the surface ECG, the P-waves are upright (though in this case very small) in V1 and have a sawtooth pattern in the inferior leads. The atrial activation sequence follows the 'counterclockwise' pattern illustrated in Figure 3.3b. The wavefront is detected first by the proximal CS catheter (not shown here), then by the His catheter, then by the poles of the multipolar catheter located in the high, lateral and low right atrium, in that order (long solid arrow). The distal coronary sinus is activated very late. The wavefront is markedly delayed between the low right atrium and its arrival at the His location (dashed arrow); during this time it passes through the zone of slow conduction in the isthmus before ascending the septum again.

In this patient, the distal poles of the multipolar catheter — in the low right atrium — are straddling the crista terminalis. They record double atrial potentials (arrowed); in addition to the main potential, the smaller, earlier signal comes from the ascending wavefront spreading across the posterior right atrium to reach the crista terminalis.

HRA = high right atrium (poles 17–18 on Figure 3.3b)
HLRA = high lateral right atrium (poles 13–14)
LLRA = low lateral right atrium (poles 7–8)
LRA = low right atrium (poles 3–4)

Atrial flutter is in many ways an electrophysiological prototype. It was the first arrhythmia to be modeled experimentally — firstly in invertebrate tissue, then in mammalian models — and it was the first clinical arrhythmia in which a reentrant mechanism was proved by entrainment. This is an electrophysiological technique in which pacing is used to continuously reset a reentrant circuit.

Figure 3.4a illustrates the substrate for a conceptualized reentrant circuit, in which a wavefront rotates around an inexcitable obstacle. This obstacle may be an anatomical feature, such as a valve or great vessel orifice. It may be a zone that is maintained in a functionally refractory state by constant bombardment from the reentrant circuit itself. In many cases, such as typical atrial flutter, the central inexcitable zone obstacle is a combination of anatomical obstacles (tricuspid valve, venae cavae) and functional block (along the crista terminalis).

The second component of the substrate for the circuit is a zone of slow conduction. This slows the impulse sufficiently that it does not 'catch up' with the refractory tail of the preceding wave.

The left of the figure illustrates activation during normal (sinus) or paced rhythm. The right illustrates activation during reentrant tachycardia. Cardiac activation is different in the two rhythms; during paced rhythm, overall activation spreads away from the pacing site (blue arrows), while during tachycardia activation spreads out from the circuit (yellow arrows). This distinction is manifest in the different P-waves seen during paced rhythm and atrial flutter.

As shown in Figure 3.4b, a premature impulse from outside (⊓) can invade the tachycardia circuit, if it arrives with the correct timing. The impulse divides in two. In the antidromic direction (opposite to that of the circuit), it collides with, and extinguishes, the reentrant wavefront (X). In the orthodromic direction (the same as that of the circuit), it creates a new wavefront (Y), propagating round the circuit earlier than would normally have been the case. In effect, the circuit has been advanced or 'reset'.

If a continuous pacing train is now delivered, slightly faster than the tachycardia cycle length, each paced impulse advances the circuit. This continuous resetting is called entrainment.

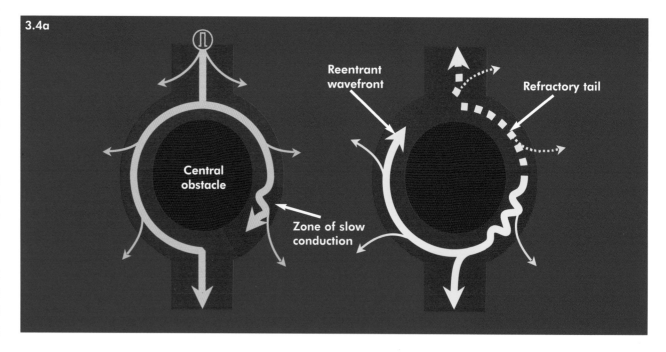

3.4a

Demonstration of entrainment is proof that an arrhythmia is due to a reentrant circuit with an excitable gap between the tail of one wavefront and the head of the next. Any of the following three criteria is proof of entrainment.

Entrainment Criterion 1: There is constant fusion at a constant pacing rate, and the last paced beat is entrained but not fused.

During entrainment, the pattern of cardiac activation (the P-wave in atrial flutter) is neither that with pacing alone (Figure 3.4a, left), nor in tachycardia alone (Figure 3.4a, right), but a fusion of the two (Figure 3.4b, left). When pacing is stopped, the last paced beat is early (i.e. entrained, like the previous paced beats) but propagates round the circuit, giving an activation pattern like the spontaneous arrhythmia (i.e. not fused; Figure 3.4b, right).

Entrainment Criterion 2: There is progressive fusion as the pacing rate increases.

If the pacing cycle length is only slightly shorter than that of the tachycardia, there is minimal invasion of the circuit (Figure 3.4c, left), and activation is similar to that by the spontaneous tachycardia — there is minimal fusion. If the pacing cycle length is progressively shortened, the circuit is invaded to a greater extent (Figure 3.4c, right). As fusion increases, cardiac activation progressively comes to resemble that seen during pacing alone.

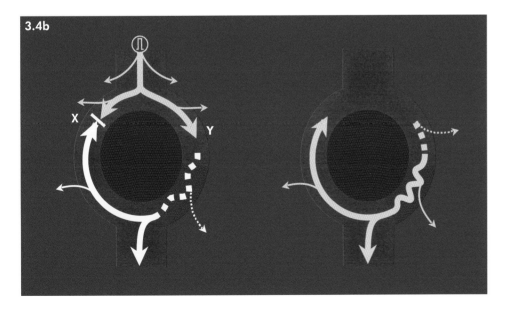

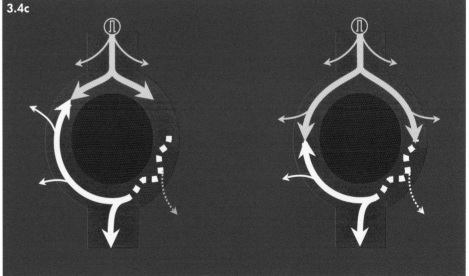

Entrainment Criterion 3: Tachycardia interruption is accompanied by block to a recording site, followed by activation of the same site from a different direction.

In Figure 3.4d, recording site R is located near the exit of the zone of slow conduction. Left: during tachycardia, it is activated by a wavefront (yellow) emerging from this zone, traveling from right to left in the figure. The next paced beat (blue) is too premature to propagate; it collides with both the head (X) and refractory tail (Y) of its predecessor, and it fails to conduct to R. Center: the next beat is purely paced, and R is activated from the opposite direction. Right: if this was a case in which the central obstacle was a zone of functional block caused by the tachycardia (see earlier), the purely paced impulses may now traverse this zone, activating R from a different direction altogether.

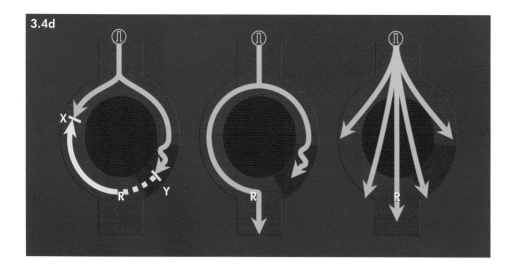

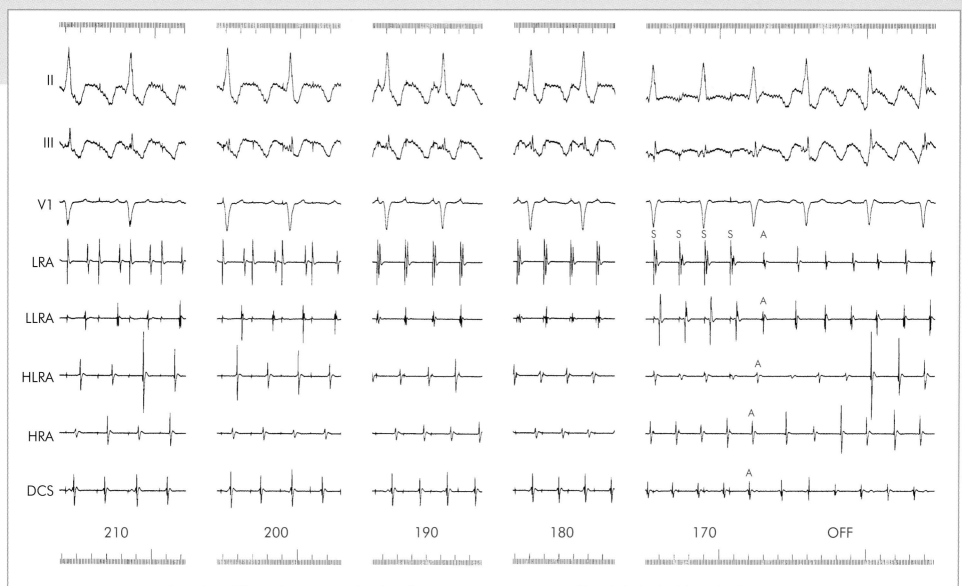

Tracing 3.4 Entrainment of typical atrial flutter. This tracing is taken from the same patient as Tracing 3.3 (although the leads of the multipolar catheter are displayed in the reverse order). Incremental pacing (cycle lengths displayed at the bottom) is performed using a catheter (not shown) in the low lateral right atrium. The surface P-wave morphology is stable at each cycle length. As the pacing cycle length is decreased, however, the morphology gradually shifts from that of spontaneous arrhythmia to one resembling a purely paced rhythm. On the far right, pacing is stopped, revealing the spontaneous arrhythmia. Thus, the tracing demonstrates both constant fusion at a constant paced rate and progressive fusion with an increasing paced rate. The last entrained cycle after pacing has the activation sequence of the tachycardia (A-A-A-A-A), rather than that of previous entrained cycles. Thus, entrainment criterion 1 is satisfied (though unfortunately the P-wave is obscured by a QRS complex).

3.5A TYPICAL ATRIAL FLUTTER

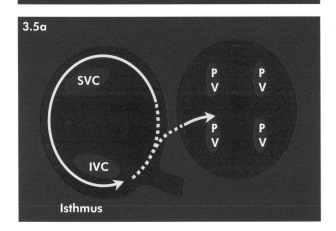

3.5a

Typical atrial flutter is by far the most frequent fast (>200 beats/min) regular atrial tachycardia. Viewed from the cardiac apex, the right atrium is activated in a counterclockwise direction.

Recent observations have established the mechanisms of a number of other macro-reentrant atrial arrhythmias, all of which have been called atypical atrial flutter.

3.5B 'CLOCKWISE' ATRIAL FLUTTER

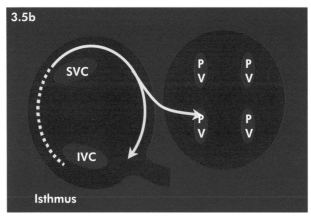

3.5b

The most frequent of these variants appears to be 'clockwise' atrial flutter. This arrhythmia is suggested on the surface ECG by notched, upright P-waves in the inferior leads and inverted P-waves in lead V1. The cycle length is similar to that of typical flutter, and intracardiac electrograms demonstrate that the reentrant circuit follows the same path, but in the opposite direction. The importance of recognizing this arrhythmia is that, like typical flutter, it is 'isthmus-dependent'. This means that the flutter circuit has to pass through the isthmus of tissue between the tricuspid annulus and the inferior vena cava, and can be treated by ablation of this isthmus (see Section 8).

3.5C TRUE ATYPICAL FLUTTER

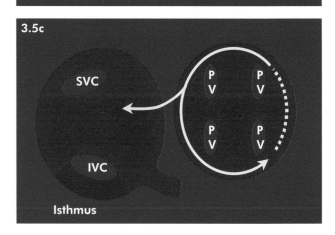

3.5c

Truly atypical flutter has a variety of ECG manifestations, and tends to have a shorter cycle length and be less stable than typical flutter and its clockwise variant. Transitions to and from atrial fibrillation are frequent. Mapping studies have suggested that a variety of circuits are possible, such as one around the pulmonary veins.

3.5D   SCAR-RELATED FLUTTER

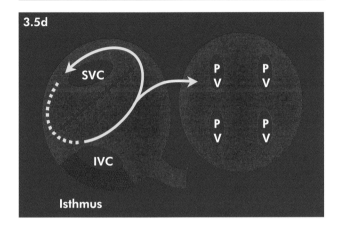

A special case is flutter caused by a circuit turning around a scar from a previous atriotomy or an atrial patch or baffle. This is particularly common following surgery for congenital heart disease. Atypical and scar-related flutter are not generally isthmus-dependent.

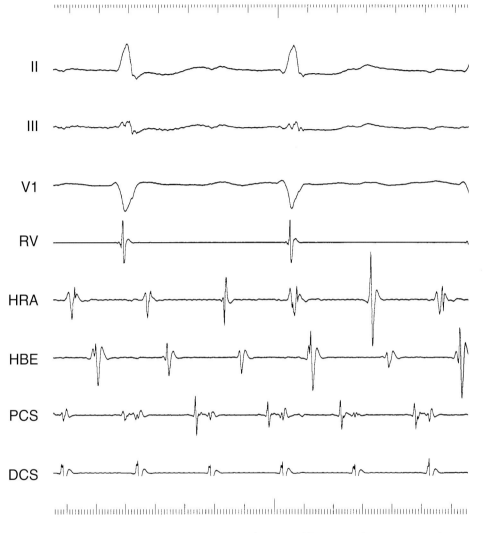

Tracing 3.5 Atypical atrial flutter (cycle length 250 ms) with a variable ventricular response. The P-waves are ill defined and the sawtooth pattern is absent in the inferior leads (compare with Tracing 3.3). The arrhythmia has been slowed considerably by oral amiodarone therapy; the majority of atypical atrial flutters have a cycle length <200 ms. The His catheter has been pulled back slightly to emphasize atrial activation. This arrhythmia could be induced, entrained and terminated by right atrial pacing. It is not possible to determine the path of this flutter circuit from the tracing shown, but it is clearly not that of typical counterclockwise flutter, as in this case His activation follows that of the high right atrium.

Atrial fibrillation (AF) is characterized on the surface ECG by irregularly irregular RR intervals, with no discernible organized P-waves. Our understanding of the electrophysiological mechanisms underlying AF is changing rapidly. The arrhythmia was originally thought to be caused by multiple atrial ectopic foci.

3.6A MULTIPLE WAVELET MODEL

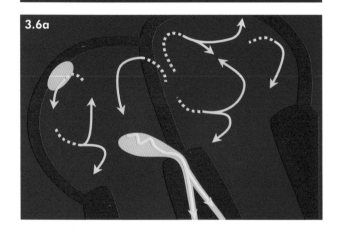

3.6a

In the last two decades, an alternative model has dominated, in which multiple wavelets of depolarization propagate within the atria. These can divide, coalesce and extinguish each other as they travel in an apparently random fashion, seeking tissue that is excitable. This model was originally developed mathematically, then shown to be possible in animal experiments. Recent studies in patients undergoing surgery show patterns of activation resembling these multiple wavelet models. For AF to be self-sustaining, there must be sufficient space for several (usually six or more) wavelets to coexist. This is only possible if the area of inexcitable tissue behind each wavefront is sufficiently small. AF is therefore favored by slow conduction and rapid recovery of the tissue (a short refractory period). Atrial enlargement also favors AF, by increasing the surface area available for the wavelets.

3.6B FOCAL MODEL

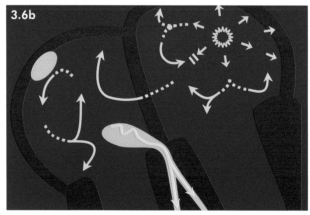

3.6b

Another hypothesis is that AF is not purely self-sustaining, but driven by a more or less stable focus or reentrant circuit. The activation arising from this focus is too rapid to be conducted uniformly throughout the atria (as in atrial tachycardia or flutter) and propagation of the wavefronts therefore breaks up into irregular wavelets — 'fibrillatory conduction' of focal or reentrant activity.

We shall not enter into the debate between proponents of the pure 'multiple wavelet' hypothesis and those who believe that AF has a focal cause. Both mechanisms can exist in animal models and it seems likely that both can exist in patients, too — possibly even at different times in the same patient. In young patients with structurally normal hearts, AF is frequently initiated (and may be perpetuated) by focal activity arising from venous structures, especially the muscular sleeves surrounding the pulmonary veins.

AF is diagnosed from a surface ECG appearance, but this appears to be a manifestation of more than one electrophysiological mechanism. Improved correlations between the clinical patterns, surface ECG, intracardiac appearances and the mechanisms of AF are needed to improve our ability to treat this condition in the EP laboratory.

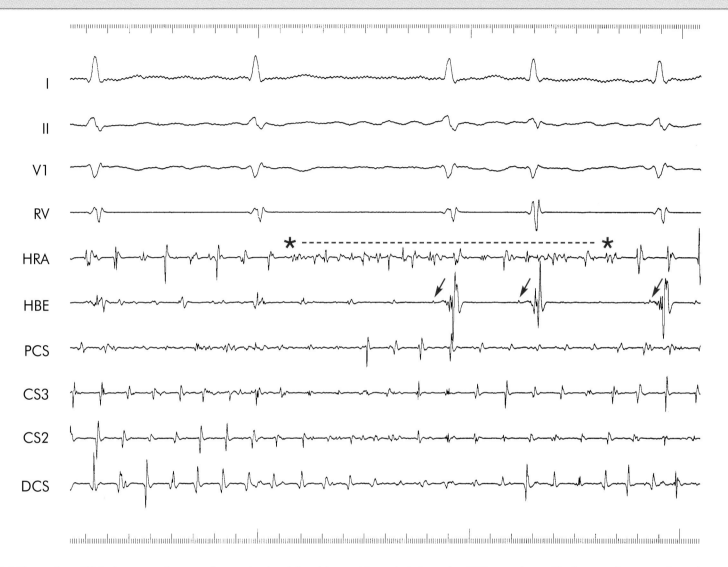

Tracing 3.6 The surface ECG shows an absence of organized atrial activity, and irregularly irregular QRS complexes. The intracardiac recordings show rapid atrial activity, which appears chaotic in some places, such as the asterisked segment in the high right atrium. However, the activation appears quite organized elsewhere; although the amplitude varies, the activation recorded by the distal coronary sinus electrodes is quite regular, with a cycle length of approximately 150 ms. Such regular activity could be taken as possible evidence of a focus or reentrant circuit that is 'driving' the AF. Conversely, it could also be that the AF is self-sustained (as in the multiple wavelet hypothesis), with a variable degree of organization dictated by local anatomical and functional features. Note that in the second half of the tracing, the His catheter records very small atrial deflections with a small His deflection (arrowed) prior to each ventricular electrogram. Even during AF, a His bundle electrogram can very often be located.

FURTHER READING

1. Olgin JE. Sinus tachycardia and sinus node reentry. In: Zipes DP, Jalife J. Cardiac Electrophysiology: From Cell to Bedside. Philadelphia: WB Saunders, 1999:459–67.

2. Krahn AD, Yee R, Klein GJ et al. Inappropriate sinus tachycardia: evaluation and therapy. J Cardiovasc Electrophysiol 1995;6(12):1124–8.

3. Lee RJ, Kalman JM, Fitzpatrick AP et al. Radiofrequency catheter modification of the sinus node for 'inappropriate' sinus tachycardia. Circulation 1995;92(10):2919–28.

4. Chen SA, Tai CT, Chiang CE et al. Focal atrial tachycardia: reanalysis of the clinical and electrophysiologic characteristics and prediction of successful radiofrequency ablation. J Cardiovasc Electrophysiol 1998;9(4):355–65.

5. Olgin JE, Lesh MD. The laboratory evaluation and role of catheter ablation for patients with atrial flutter. Cardiol Clin 1997;15(4):677–88.

6. Kalman JM, Olgin JE, Saxon LA et al. Electrocardiographic and electrophysiologic characterization of atypical atrial flutter in man: use of activation and entrainment mapping and implications for catheter ablation. J Cardiovasc Electrophysiol 1997;8(2):121–44.

7. Levy S, Breithardt G, Campbell RW et al. Atrial fibrillation: current knowledge and recommendations for management. Working Group on Arrhythmias of the European Society of Cardiology. Eur Heart J 1998;19(9):1294–320.

8. Allessie MA, Konings K, Kirchhof CJ et al. Electrophysiologic mechanisms of perpetuation of atrial fibrillation. Am J Cardiol 1996;77(3):10A–23A.

9. Haissaguerre M, Jais P, Shah DC et al. Spontaneous initiation of atrial fibrillation by ectopic beats originating in the pulmonary veins. N Engl J Med 1998;339(10):659–66.

Atrioventricular nodal reentrant tachycardia (AVNRT) is the most common arrhythmia that is routinely amenable to catheter ablation, and accounts for around 25% of the cases presenting to our electrophysiology (EP) laboratories.

Although the principles of dual AV nodal pathways and AVNRT have been understood for more than 25 years, the anatomical correlates of the fast and slow 'pathways' have only recently become clear. It was originally thought that AVNRT was caused by micro-reentry entirely within the AV node. However, surgical and, later, catheter ablation have demonstrated that the fast and slow pathways actually represent anatomically distinct atrial inputs to the compact AV node. A considerable portion of the AVNRT circuit is within the right atrium and reentry can therefore be interrupted by ablation without injury to the compact AV node itself.

This section describes the electrophysiological and anatomical bases of dual AV nodal pathways, together with the mechanisms of typical AV nodal reentry and its variants. Methods used to differentiate AVNRT from other supraventricular tachycardias will be discussed in Section 6. The principles of catheter ablation for AV nodal reentry will be described in Section 8.

In many patients, there appear to be at least two discrete inputs from the atria to the AV node. These are commonly termed the fast and slow 'pathways'. In fast sinus rhythm, the fast pathway (FP) constitutes the normal entry of the atrial impulse into the compact AV node. Although careful electrophysiological testing may demonstrate the presence of a slow pathway (SP) in up to one-third of patients, it is probably not relevant to normal conduction.

4.1A   FAST PATHWAY

Usually, conduction through the AV node is via the fast pathway. The normal characteristics of the AV node, described in Section 2, are actually those of fast-pathway conduction. Conduction down the slow pathway (wavy line, Figure 4.1a) is usually blocked in the node at the point where the two pathways join, as that tissue is still recovering from depolarization via the fast pathway.

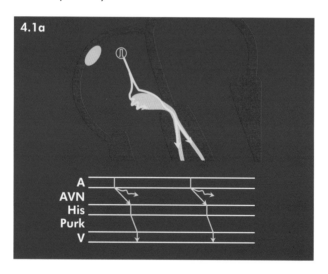

4.1a

4.1B   SLOW PATHWAY

An early atrial extrastimulus may be blocked in the fast pathway, yet still conduct down a slow pathway. This is because the slow pathway has a shorter effective refractory period (ERP). Because it is now using the slow pathway, the impulse takes longer to travel through the node, and the AH interval is consequently prolonged.

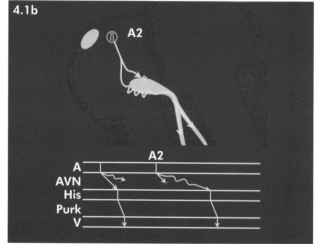

4.1b

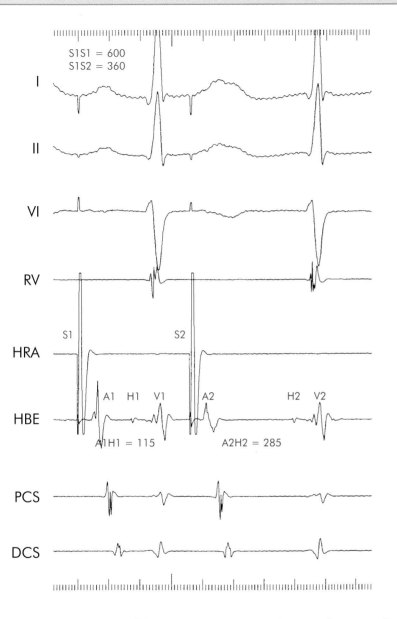

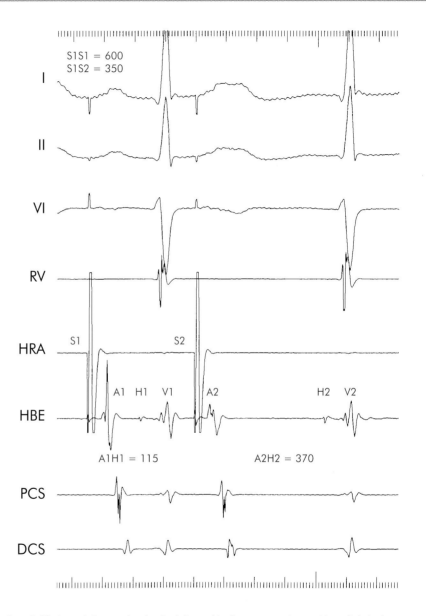

Tracing 4.1a Following an atrial drive train (S1S1 = 600 ms), an atrial extrastimulus is given (S1S2 = 360 ms). The AH interval of the extrastimulus (A2H2) is greater than that of the drive train (A1H1) because of decrement in the AV node.

Tracing 4.1b An atrial extrastimulus is delivered in the same patient, with a slightly shorter coupling interval (S1S1 = 600 ms, S1S2 = 350 ms). The A1A2 is less than the ERP of the fast pathway, which blocks, and the impulse can now only conduct down the slow pathway. The AH interval of the extrastimulus increases from 285 to 370 ms, a 'jump' of 85 ms.

4.1C A-H JUMP

The appearance of dual AV nodal pathways on the antegrade conduction curve is shown. With increasingly premature atrial complexes (decreasing A1A2 on the x-axis), the ERP of the fast pathway is reached, and the impulse can now only conduct down the slow pathway. At this point, an abrupt increase is seen in the length of the AH interval; this is termed an A-H jump.

A jump is classically defined as an increase in the length of the AH interval of ≥50 ms, caused by a decrease in the coupling interval of an atrial extrastimulus (A1A2) of 10 ms. Even if these criteria are not formally met, dual AV nodal physiology can be inferred from the presence of discontinuity in the conduction curves, with two clearly discrete sections. Furthermore, dual AV nodal pathways and AVNRT can exist with little or no discrete jump, as the slow- and fast-pathway portions of the curve may lie close together. In rare cases, the presence of more than one discontinuity of the AV node conduction curve suggests the presence of multiple AV nodal 'pathways'.

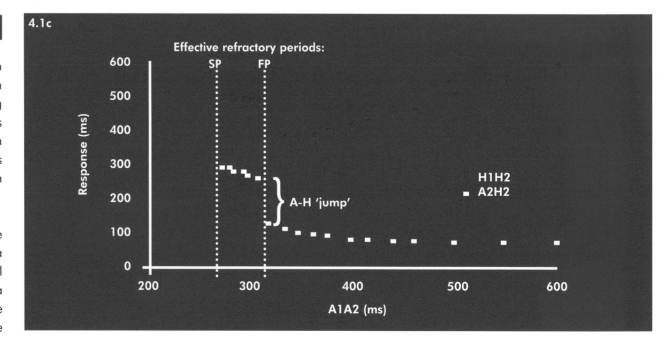

4.1c

4.1D 'TWO-FOR-ONE' RESPONSE

In patients with dual pathways, the AV nodal tissue occasionally has time to recover between fast and slow pathway conduction. From time-to-time, a single atrial impulse causes two His-ventricular depolarizations. This 'two-for-one' phenomenon is quite rare.

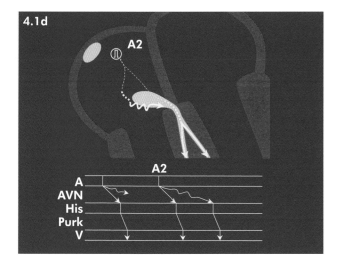

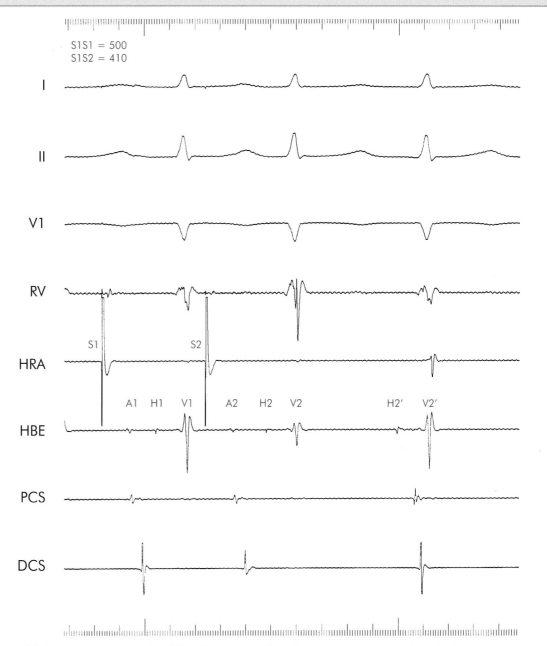

Tracing 4.1d An atrial extrastimulus (S2) gives rise to a 'two-for-one' response: the impulse is conducted through the node down both the fast pathway (H2, V2) and the slow pathway (H2', V2'). The second response gives rise to an atrial 'echo' cycle (see next section).

4.2A TYPICAL AV NODAL ECHO

If the premature impulse is delayed sufficiently as it travels down the slow pathway of the AV node, the fast pathway may recover its excitability and conduct the impulse back to the atria. This is an atrial 'echo' cycle, due to AV reentry in the AV node, commonly referred to as an 'AV nodal echo' though this term is not strictly correct. Because the impulse returns up the fast pathway at the same time as it is traveling down the His-Purkinje system, ventricular and atrial activation are virtually simultaneous. AV nodal echo beats confirm that dual AV nodal pathways are present and also that the fast pathway can conduct in a retrograde direction.

4.2B INITIATION OF AVNRT

If the slow pathway is no longer refractory by the time the impulse has returned to the atrium, repeat conduction down it may occur, and the first cycle of AVNRT is initiated.

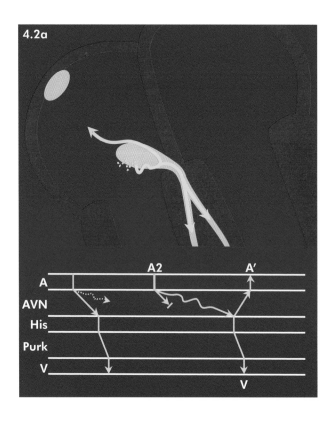

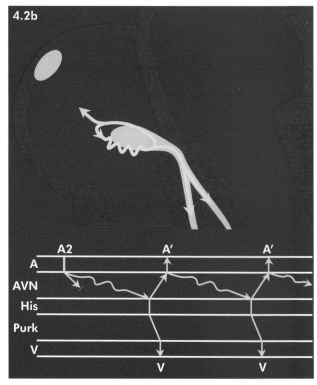

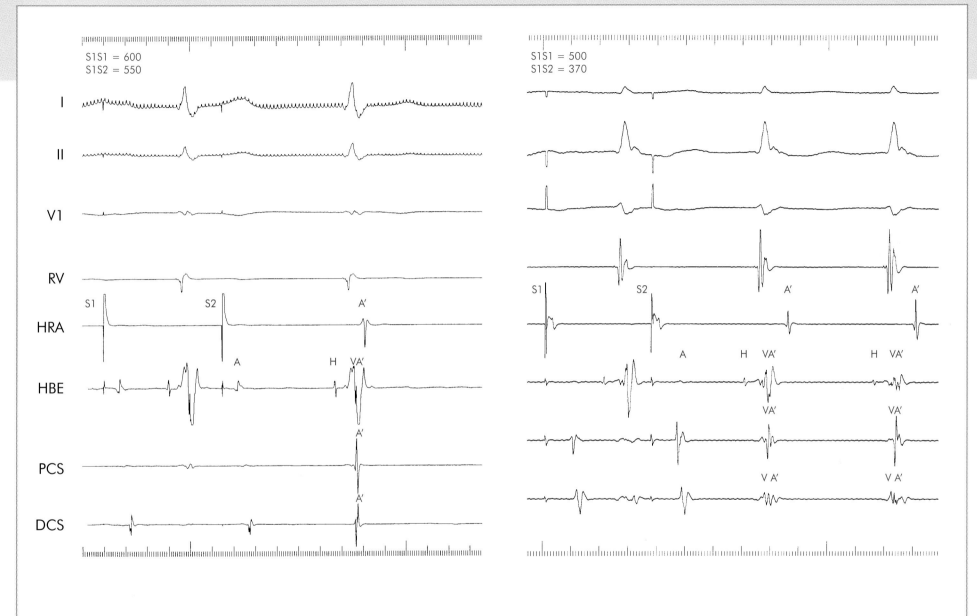

Tracing 4.2a An atrial premature complex (S2) is conducted down the slow pathway and returns up the fast pathway to produce an echo (A'), which is virtually simultaneous with the ventricular electrogram.

Tracing 4.2b S2 is again conducted down the slow pathway and returns up the fast pathway. On this occasion, the echo beat (A') finds the slow pathway to be excitable and AVNRT is induced.

In patients with retrograde conduction, a 'jump' in the VA interval may be seen with progressively premature ventricular extrastimuli. This may be due to dual retrograde AV nodal pathways (the counterpart of the antegrade jump described in Section 4.1), or to the onset of delay in the His-Purkinje system.

4.3A   DUAL RETROGRADE AV NODAL PATHWAYS

At long coupling intervals, ventricular extrastimuli are conducted up the His-Purkinje system and exit the node via the fast pathway to the atria. With progressive prematurity, smooth decremental conduction usually occurs in the VA interval. In the presence of dual retrograde AV nodal pathways, a jump in VA interval may occur as the fast pathway of the AV node blocks, allowing conduction up the slow pathway to the atria. Sometimes this is followed by an 'atypical' echo back over the fast pathway.

4.3B   VA 'JUMP' DUE TO INFRA-HIS DELAY

Progressive prematurity of ventricular extrastimuli may also cause a sudden increase in VA interval due to block in the His-Purkinje system below the AV node. In the diagram, retrograde block has occurred in the right bundle branch, so the impulse has to travel across the interventricular septum and reach the His bundle via the left bundle branch. This delay may reveal a retrograde His potential, which is normally buried within the ventricular electrogram. In our experience, jumps in VA conduction are more commonly due to infra-His block than dual retrograde AV nodal pathways.

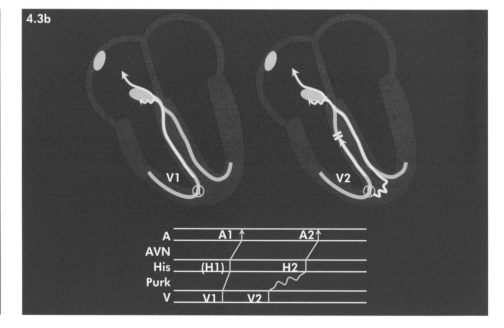

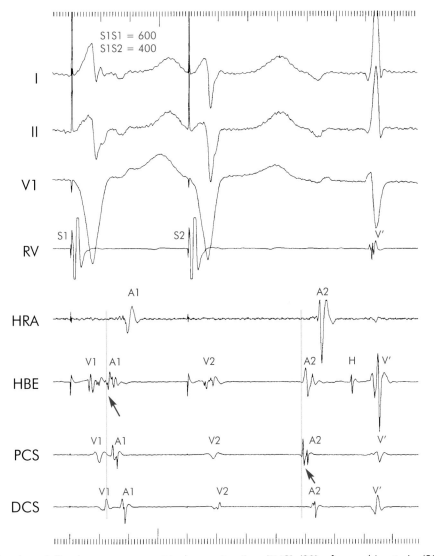

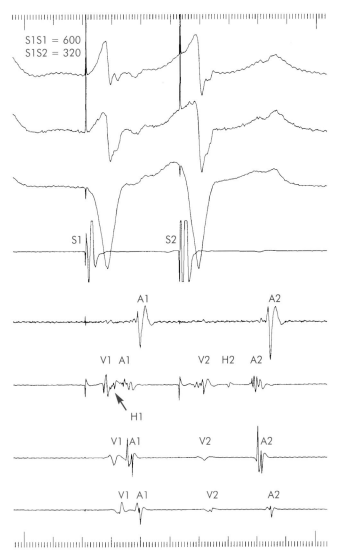

Tracing 4.3a A premature ventricular contraction (PVC) (S2) after a drive train (S1) causes a retrograde jump — there is a marked increase in VA interval as the impulse conducts solely up the slow pathway. Note that the atrial activation is now recorded slightly earlier by the PCS catheter (arrow, cursor) than the His catheter, as the former is closer to the slow pathway exit site (see Section 4.4). By the time the right atrium is reached, the fast pathway is no longer refractory and the impulse can travel down it, causing an 'atypical' echo beat (V').

Tracing 4.3b A retrograde His potential (H1, H2) moves out considerably after the ventricular extrastimulus. The increase in the VA interval is largely due to a jump in V2H2, not H2A2, indicating retrograde conduction delay in the His-Purkinje system rather than the AV node.

The AV node and related structures lie along the septal portion of the tricuspid valve annulus. This region is termed the triangle of Koch, with the CS os at its base, the other two sides being the tendon of Todaro and the tricuspid annulus itself. The compact AV node and penetrating bundle of His are toward the apex of the triangle.

4.4A　LOCATION OF THE FAST AND SLOW 'PATHWAYS'

Surgical and catheter ablation experience indicates that, in the majority of patients, the 'fast pathway' appears to be atrial tissue situated anterosuperior to the compact AV node, while the 'slow pathway' appears to be a zone of atrial tissue along the tricuspid annulus posteroinferior to the node. The nature of these 'pathways' is the subject of speculation; one view is that they are not discrete tracts but atrial tissue forming functionally separate inputs to the node. However, posterior extensions of AV nodal tissue have been described which may themselves constitute the 'slow pathway'.

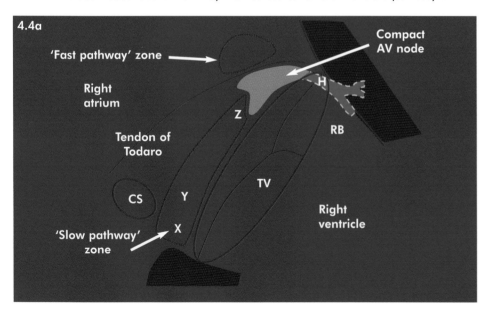

4.4B　POTENTIALS RECORDED IN THE REGION OF THE AV NODE

A mapping catheter exploring the posterior part of the triangle of Koch can often record potentials that are separate from both the local atrial electrogram and the His potential (H in Figure 4.4a). These have been termed 'slow pathway' (SP) potentials, but their exact cause is unclear. Near the CS os (X), the atrial electrogram may be sharp but the SP potential may be of low frequency and amplitude. At a slightly more anterior location (Y) the SP potential may become more discrete, even if smaller, and the atrial electrogram may become less well defined. At an even more anterior location (Z), neither the SP nor the His potential can be recorded; this is the approximate location of the AV node. If the catheter is advanced beyond the His location, a right bundle branch (RBB) potential can often be recorded (Tracing 4.4b).

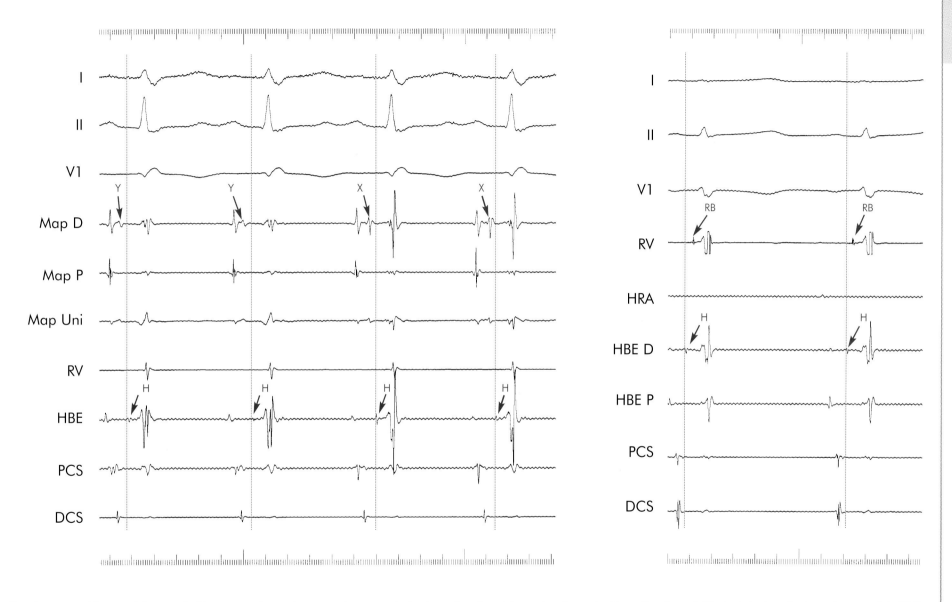

Tracing 4.4a SP potentials recorded by a mapping catheter moving posteriorly along the tricuspid annulus, from site Y to site X. Note that the SP potentials are earlier than the His potentials (arrows and cursors). SP potentials as clear as these are extremely unusual.

Tracing 4.4b A right bundle branch potential (RBB) recorded by a mapping catheter positioned beyond the His position.

AVNRT can take several forms, with a confusing variety of accompanying names. We prefer to use the term 'typical' to refer to the classical type, seen in approximately 90% of patients, and to call all other forms 'atypical'. It should be stressed that the anatomical basis of the varieties of AVNRT is not clear, and these figures are not intended to be anatomically accurate.

4.5A TYPICAL AVNRT: SLOW-FAST WITH ANTERIOR EXIT

The impulse travels down the slow pathway and returns via the fast pathway (i.e. 'slow-fast'). The earliest atrial activation is in the anterior septum, recorded by the His catheter.

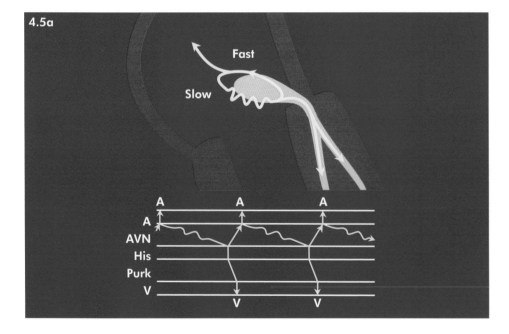

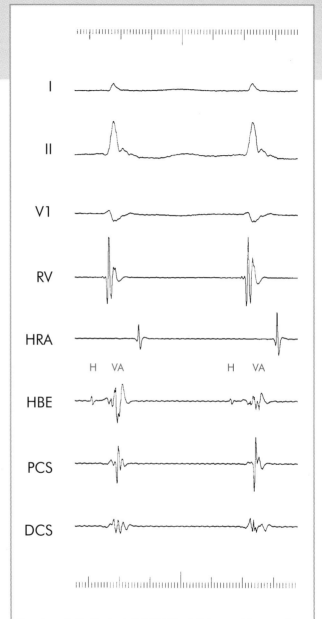

Tracing 4.5a Typical AVNRT. The VA interval is very short and the earliest atrial activation is seen in the anterior septum (recorded by the His catheter, buried in the ventricular electrogram).

4.5B ATYPICAL AVNRT: SLOW-FAST WITH POSTERIOR EXIT

In a slightly different form of slow-fast AVNRT, the atria are activated via the posterior septum, so that the earliest atrial electrogram is recorded by the proximal CS electrode. Both forms of slow-fast AVNRT have been termed 'common' AVNRT, but we believe this nomenclature may be confusing.

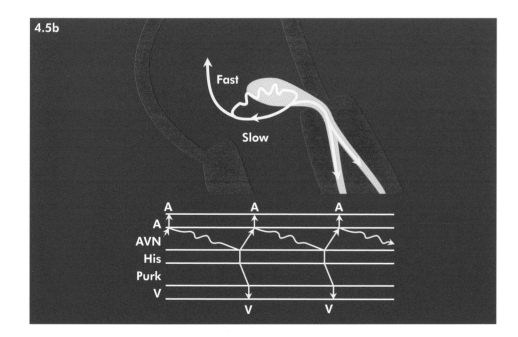

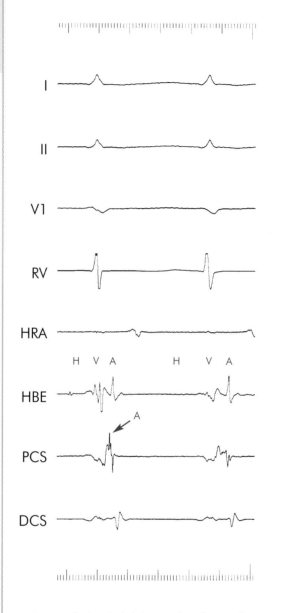

Tracing 4.5b Atypical AVNRT, 'slow-fast' with posterior exit. Again, the VA interval is very short, but this time the earliest atrial activation is recorded by the proximal CS electrode (arrow).

4.5C ATYPICAL AVNRT: 'FAST-SLOW'

This appears to be the reverse of the typical form; the impulse travels down the fast pathway and returns to the atria via the slow pathway. This is one cause of 'long RP' tachycardia (see Section 6.7).

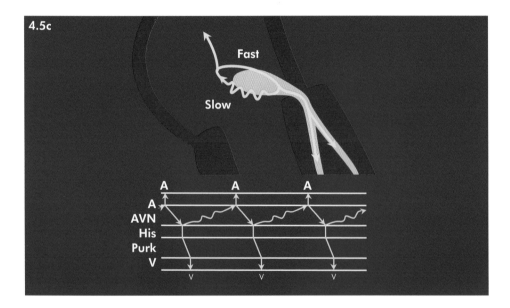

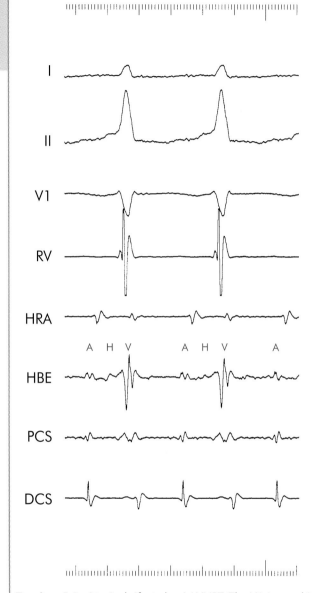

Tracing 4.5c Atypical, 'fast-slow' AVNRT. The VA interval is much longer than in typical AVNRT. The AH interval is short, and the HA' is long, indicating that antegrade activation is over the fast pathway and retrograde activation is over the slow pathway. See Tracing 6.7b for another example.

4.5D   ATYPICAL AVNRT: 'SLOW-SLOW'

This appears to use two slow pathways for the two limbs of the circuit. It is not clear whether these two limbs are anatomically distinct from each other and from the fast pathway, and if so in what way.

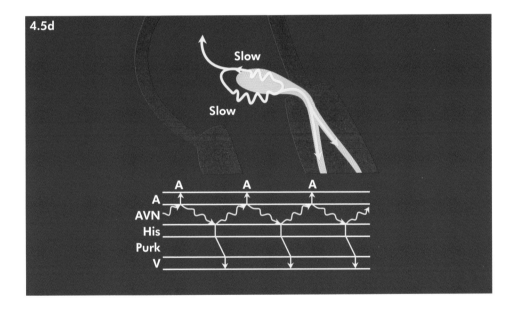

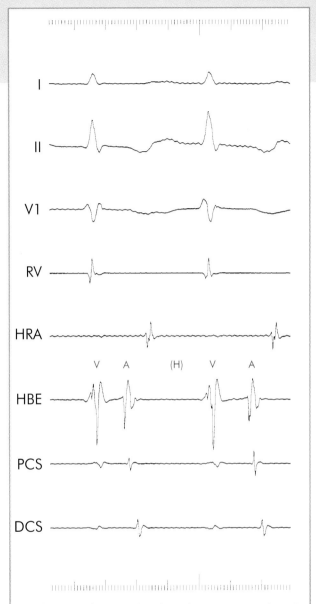

Tracing 4.5d Atypical, 'slow-slow' AVNRT. The His recording is not clear in this tracing, but inferred from elsewhere. Both the AH and HA intervals are long.

FURTHER READING

1. Cosio FG, Anderson RH, Kuck KH et al. ESCWGA/NASPE/P experts consensus statement: living anatomy of the atrioventricular junctions. A guide to electrophysiologic mapping. Working Group of Arrhythmias of the European Society of Cardiology. North American Society of Pacing and Electrophysiology. J Cardiovasc Electrophysiol 1999;10(8):1162–70.

2. AV node reentry. In: Prystowsky EN, Klein GJ. Cardiac Arrhythmias: An Integrated Approach for the Clinician. New York: McGraw-Hill, 1994:115–25.

3. Otomo K, Wang Z, Lazarra R et al. Atrioventricular nodal reentrant tachycardia: Electrophysiological characteristics of four forms and implications for the reentrant circuit. In: Zipes DP, Jalife J. Cardiac Electrophysiology: From Cell to Bedside. Philadelphia: WB Saunders, 1999:504–20.

4. Mazgalev TN, Tchou PJ, editors. Atrial-AV Nodal Electrophysiology: A View for the Millennium. Armonk New York: Futura Publishing, 2000.

ACCESSORY PATHWAYS AND AV REENTRY

5

This section discusses the anatomy, behavior and classification of accessory atrioventricular (AV) pathways. Pacing methods used in the electrophysiology (EP) laboratory to demonstrate the presence of these pathways are described, as are the initiation and appearance of atrioventricular reentrant tachycardia (AVRT). Finally, the nomenclature for rarer types of accessory pathway is discussed. The differential diagnosis of supraventricular tachycardias will be discussed in Section 6.

An accessory AV pathway can provide an alternative route for atrial activation to reach the ventricle. Depolarization of the ventricle earlier than would be expected had conduction gone only over the normal AV conduction system is termed ventricular 'pre-excitation'. During sinus rhythm or atrial pacing, the degree of ventricular pre-excitation depends on the relative times taken for the atrial impulse to reach the AV node and the pathway, and the times taken to conduct over each.

In sinus rhythm, a delta-wave may be absent either because the accessory pathway does not conduct in the antegrade direction (a 'concealed' accessory pathway), or because the atrial impulse arrives too late to contribute to ventricular activation ('latent' pre-excitation). Two maneuvers can be used to increase the pre-excitation: (1) induction of delay in the AV node; and (2) differential atrial pacing (see Section 5.5).

5.1A   MINIMAL PRE-EXCITATION

The figure shows a heart with an accessory pathway connecting the left atrium and ventricle. During right atrial pacing the impulse reaches the AV node rapidly, while it can take a long time to reach the left atrial origin of the pathway. Most of the ventricle is therefore depolarized by the His-Purkinje system and there is minimal pre-excitation.

5.1B   DELAY IN AV NODE INCREASES PRE-EXCITATION

AV nodal conduction can be slowed using drugs such as adenosine or verapamil, which do not affect the accessory pathway. Alternatively, conduction of a premature atrial stimulus (or a spontaneous atrial premature complex) may be delayed in the AV node, because of the decremental properties of the latter. This delay allows time for the greater proportion of the ventricle to be depolarized by the accessory pathway.

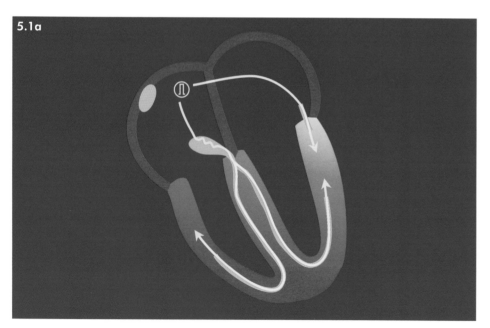

5.1a

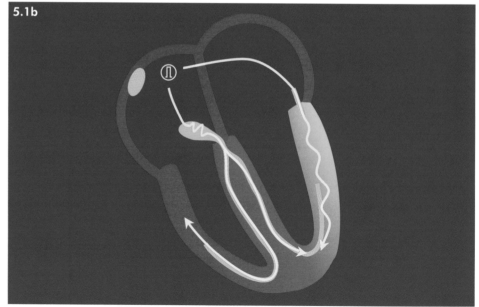

5.1b

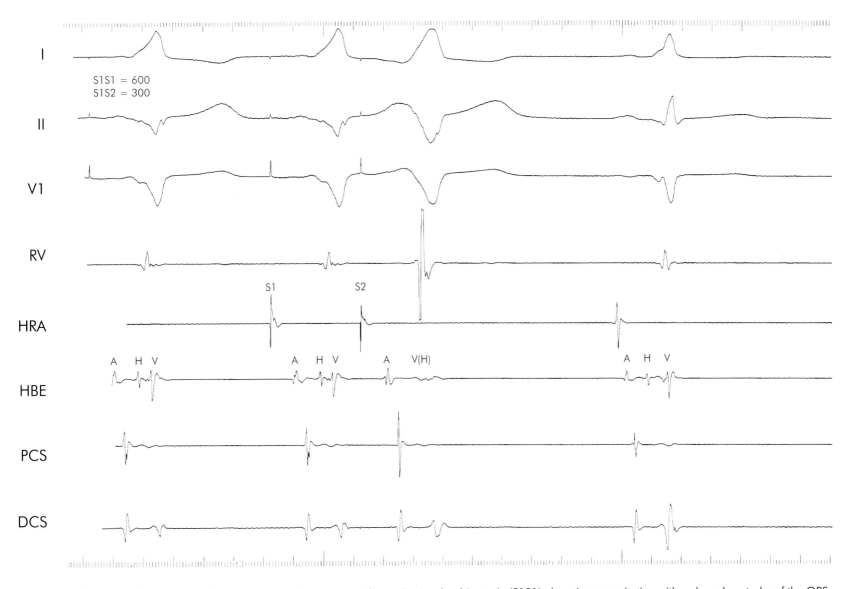

Tracing 5.1a Extrastimulus testing in a patient with a posteroseptal accessory pathway. During the drive train (S1S1), there is pre-excitation with a slurred upstroke of the QRS complex. With the extrastimulus (S2), a greater degree of pre-excitation is seen on the surface leads, because of delayed conduction through the AV node, resulting in a greater proportion of ventricular activation over the accessory pathway. The AH interval increases (the His bundle electrogram disappears into the ventricular electrogram), but the stimulus-to-delta (S-δ) interval is unchanged. The converse happens with the last beat, which is sinus in origin. The coupling interval is greater than S1S1, so conduction over the AV node is more rapid (AH is shorter) and there is less pre-excitation on the surface QRS.

5.1C   HIS EXTRASYSTOLE

Conversely, pre-excitation is minimized when atrial activation starts near the AV node and far away from the pathway, as is seen with an extrasystole arising from the AV junction. Such a beat conducts exclusively over the His-Purkinje system, and the QRS complex shows no pre-excitation. Normalization of a QRS complex with a His extrasystole is considered proof that the abnormal QRS complex is due to pre-excitation.

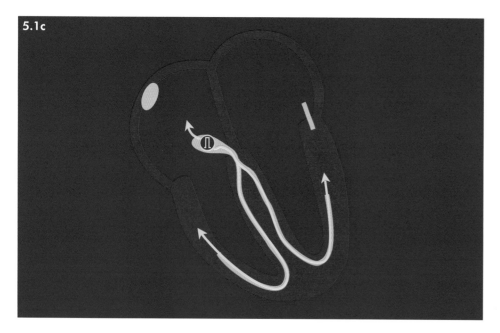

5.1c

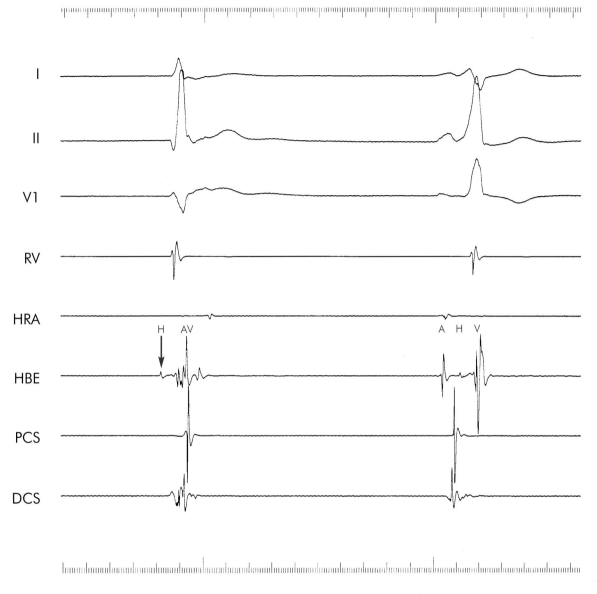

Tracing 5.1c A His extrasystole, characterized by a narrow complex QRS preceded by a His deflection (H, arrowed), which is not preceded by an atrial impulse. This impulse conducts to the ventricles exclusively over the AV node, at the same time as depolarizing the atria. The next beat is a sinus beat, which is pre-excited. This patient had a left free wall accessory pathway.

During ventricular pacing studies, the electrophysiologist is alert for changes in both the timing and pattern of atrial activation. Examination of the atrial activation sequence during ventricular pacing can give evidence of accessory pathways and their locations.

5.2A CONCENTRIC ATRIAL ACTIVATION

A patient with a left free wall accessory pathway is paced at the right ventricular apex. During a slow drive train, the atria are activated retrogradely by the AV node, as the impulse reaches the His-Purkinje system and conducts over the node before it reaches the pathway (it takes approximately 50 ms for the impulse to cross the septum to the left side). The earliest atrial activation is therefore near the node and recorded by the His bundle catheter (concentric atrial activation).

5.2B ECCENTRIC RETROGRADE ATRIAL ACTIVATION

More rapid ventricular pacing, or a ventricular extrastimulus, results in delay in retrograde conduction in the node (due to decremental conduction), so that the pathway now depolarizes the atria first. The earliest atrial activation is now in the left atrium, as recorded by the coronary sinus (CS) catheter. Retrograde atrial activation other than by the AV node is termed eccentric.

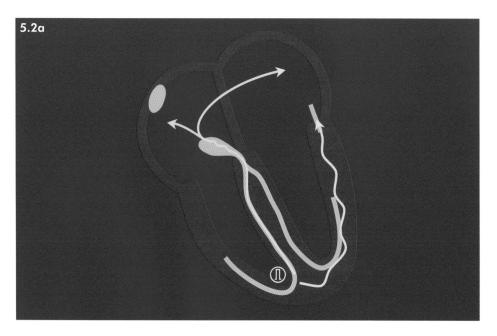

5.2a

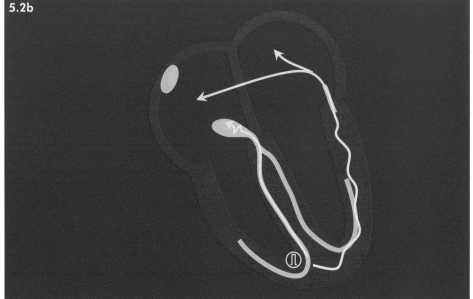

5.2b

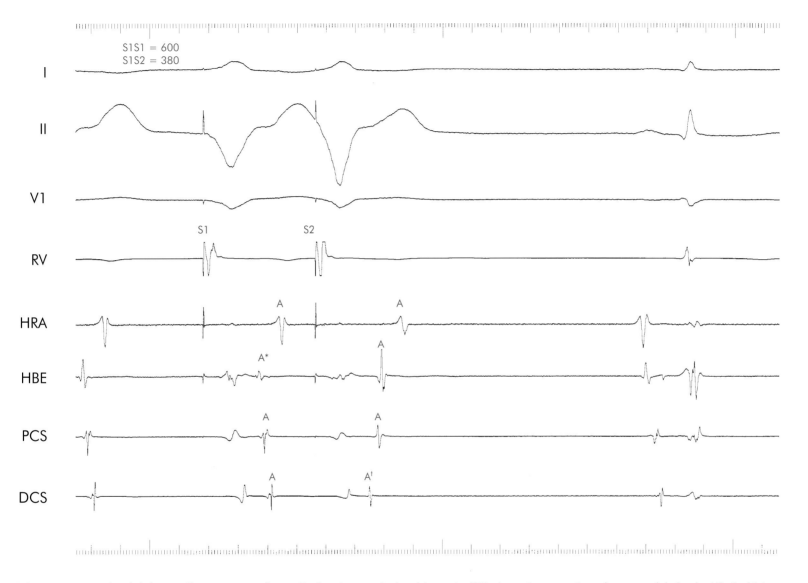

Tracing 5.2a A patient with a left free wall accessory pathway. During the ventricular drive train (S1), the atria are activated retrogradely by the His-Purkinje system and the AV node. The earliest atrial signal (A*) is recorded by the His catheter — indicating concentric atrial activation. A ventricular extrastimulus (S2) with a coupling interval of 380 ms is delayed in the AV node, allowing the impulse to travel up the pathway to the atria. Atrial activation (A2) is now eccentric, with the earliest signal (A†) recorded by the distal coronary sinus catheter.

5.2C CHANGE FROM ECCENTRIC TO CONCENTRIC ATRIAL ACTIVATION

If a ventricular extrastimulus is delivered within the refractory period of the pathway, then its conduction will be blocked in the pathway but may still slowly reach the atrium over the AV node.

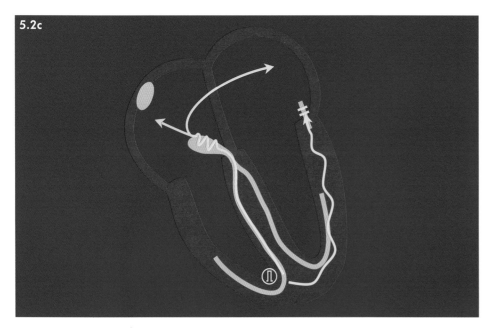

5.2c

Therefore, ventricular pacing at decreasing cycle lengths, or increasingly premature extrastimuli, may show a change in atrial activation from concentric to eccentric, or from eccentric to concentric.

In many patients, the AV node does not conduct retrogradely at all, and eccentric conduction is seen at all cycle lengths until the pathway blocks. In others, retrograde conduction in the node may be so rapid that pathway conduction is difficult to discern. Apart from ventricular pacing and premature ventricular contractions (PVCs), eccentric atrial activation can be made clearer by: (1) slowing or blocking conduction over the node with drugs such as adenosine; (2) differential ventricular pacing (pacing at a site close to the accessory pathway — see Section 5.6); or (3) observing orthodromic tachycardia, in which retrograde conduction is exclusively over the accessory pathway (see Section 5.4).

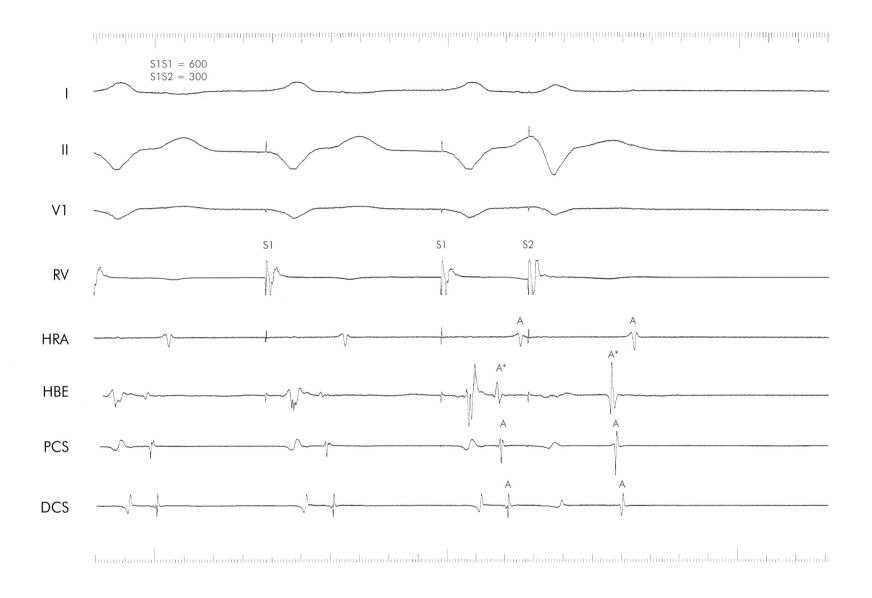

Tracing 5.2c In the same patient as Tracing 5.2a, a more closely coupled extrastimulus (S2) reaches the accessory pathway within its refractory period and is therefore blocked. The shorter refractory period of the AV node results in a concentric atrial activation pattern similar to that in the drive train (S1). Again, the earliest atrial activation is in the His bundle electrogram (A*) but there is considerable delay because of decremental conduction in the AV node.

Accessory pathways can be situated anywhere along either AV annulus, with the exception of the portion of the mitral annulus that is adjacent to the aortic valve.

5.3A   TRADITIONAL NOMENCLATURE

The figure represents the AV annuli viewed from below (equivalent to the left anterior oblique radiographic projection). The traditional nomenclature divides locations into: left anterolateral, left lateral, left posterior, right anterior, right lateral and right posterior. Septal pathways can be left- or right-sided. Posteroseptal pathways are located near the coronary sinus os; mid-septal pathways lie anterior to this (this is the closest location to the compact AV node). An anteroseptal location is one from which the His potential can be recorded.

5.3B   PROPOSED NOMENCLATURE

Although the previous classification is in widespread use, it is not strictly correct anatomically. The 'septal' regions include tissue that is not truly septal, and the 'anterior' and 'posterior' directions are actually more superior and inferior. A more correct terminology has been proposed (Figure 5.3b). However, old habits die hard, and it is not clear whether the new terminology will prevail.

AV= aortic valve, PV= pulmonary valve, MV= mitral valve, TV= tricuspid valve.

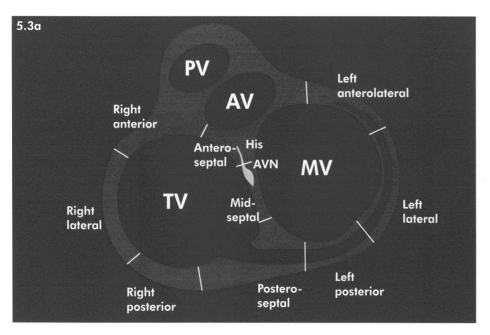

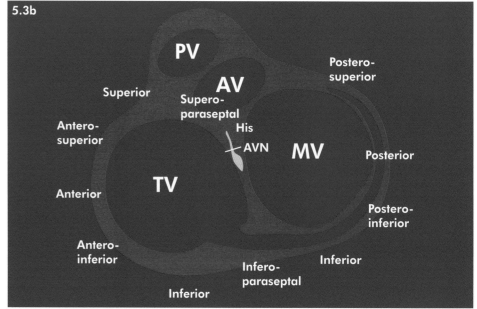

Tracings 5.3a–d show examples of retrograde conduction by pathways in different locations. In each case, S1 is the last beat of a ventricular drive train. S2 is a ventricular extrastimulus that conducts up the pathway because of delay or block in the node.

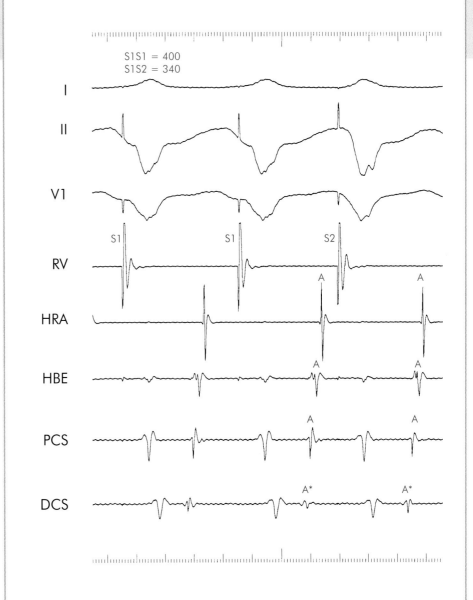

Tracing 5.3a Left lateral pathway. The earliest atrial activation (A*) is recorded at the distal CS, both during the drive train and after the extrastimulus.

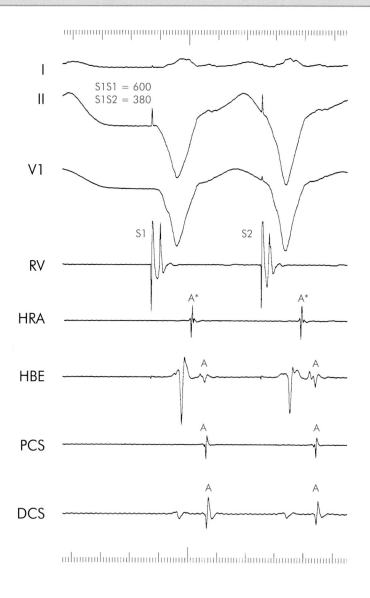

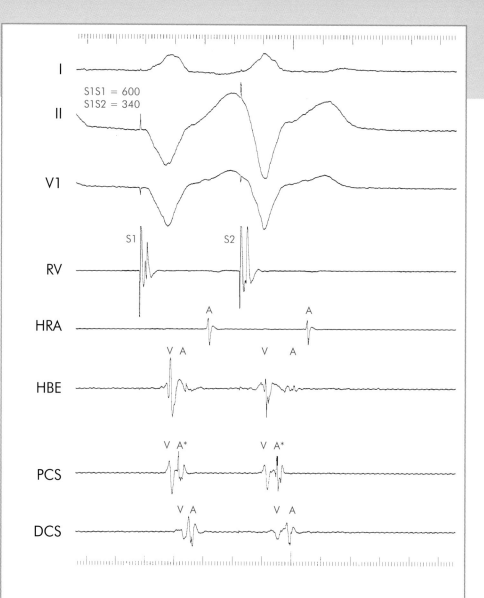

Tracing 5.3b Right free wall pathway. There is no electrode on the tricuspid annulus near the pathway, but right atrial activation (A*) is much earlier at the HRA catheter than at the His position or in the CS. This indicates eccentric atrial activation due to a right-sided accessory pathway (but should also prompt the electrophysiologist to check that the catheters have not moved!).

Tracing 5.3c Posteroseptal pathway. The earliest atrial activation (A*) after S2 is in the proximal CS. Note that the atrial activation recorded at the His catheter is almost as early as that in the proximal CS following S1, but that after S2 it is delayed due to delay in the node, making the atrial activation more eccentric. This usually represents an accessory pathway but may also be caused by a posterior retrograde exit site from the AV node (see Sections 4.3 and 4.4).

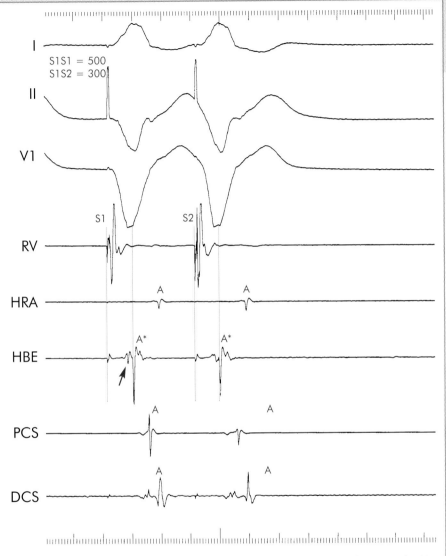

Tracing 5.3d Anteroseptal pathway. The pathway is located adjacent to the AV node. The stimulus-to-A interval recorded at the His bundle electrode is identical following S1 and S2. The lack of decrement in conduction, even with a very short V1V2 interval, suggests the possibility of an accessory pathway, which can be confirmed by other means (see Section 5.7). The early deflection (arrowed) recorded by the His bundle electrode following S1 is probably a retrograde His electrogram. It disappears into the atrial electrogram following S2, probably due to retrograde delay or block in the His-Purkinje system.

The typical initiation of AVRT by atrial extrastimuli is mechanistically analogous to that of AV nodal reentrant tachycardia (AVNRT): antegrade block in one limb of the circuit allows the impulse to turn around and activate that limb retrogradely.

5.4A   SINUS RHYTHM

In sinus rhythm, the impulse is conducted over both the AV node and the accessory pathway. As described in Section 5.1, the degree of ventricular pre-excitation depends on the relative timing of conduction over the AV node and pathway.

5.4B   PREMATURE ATRIAL COMPLEX

A premature atrial complex reaches the pathway when it is refractory and its conduction is therefore blocked. However, it conducts over the AV node and the ventricle is depolarized, this time without pre-excitation.

5.4C   INITIATION OF ORTHODROMIC AVRT

The impulse is delayed sufficiently in conducting over the AV node and ventricle so that, by the time it reaches the ventricular insertion of the accessory pathway, the latter is no longer refractory. The impulse can therefore return over the pathway, activating the atria eccentrically.

The first beat of AVRT is complete, and the circuit continues by conduction to the ventricles via the AV node once again. AVRT in which conduction over the AV node/His bundle is antegrade is termed *orthodromic* AVRT, and is by far the most common variant. An AVRT circuit can occasionally function in reverse — an example of *antidromic* tachycardia (defined as a tachycardia in which AV node/His bundle activation is retrograde) is discussed in Section 6.8.

5.4a

5.4b

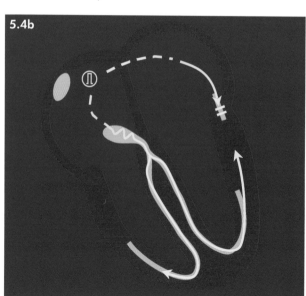

5.4c

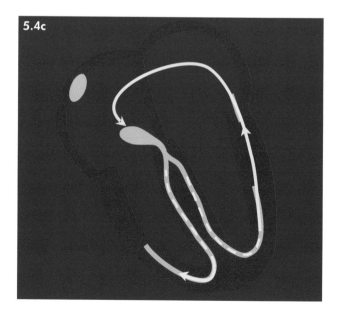

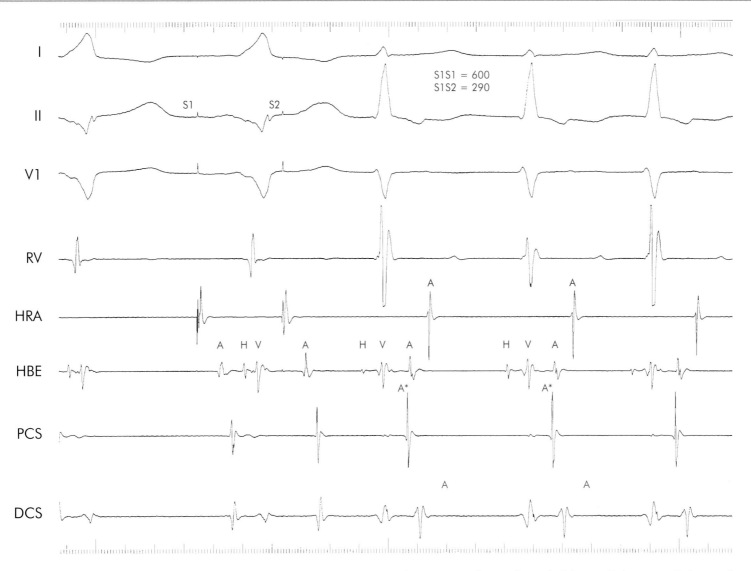

Tracing 5.4 Classical initiation of AVRT by an atrial extrastimulus in a patient with a posteroseptal accessory pathway. The end of the atrial drive train (S1) is conducted to the ventricle with pre-excitation. The atrial extrastimulus (S2) is blocked in the accessory pathway but conducts over the AV node, as the latter has the shorter refractory period. The impulse travels down the AV node and activates the entire ventricle via the His-Purkinje system, so the resulting surface QRS complex is not pre-excited. By the time the impulse reaches the accessory pathway, it is excitable and conducts the impulse in a retrograde fashion, activating the atria eccentrically (A*, recorded earliest by the proximal CS). The first cycle of the circuit is complete when the impulse returns to the right atrium. The orthodromic circuit continues with ventricular activation via the AV node (again giving a normal QRS complex) and returns over the pathway (again giving eccentric retrograde atrial activation).

Pacing at different atrial locations can be used to make pre-excitation manifest and to aid localization of the accessory pathway. With conventional high right atrial pacing, right-sided and septal accessory pathways are usually associated with overt pre-excitation because of the proximity of the pacing impulse to the accessory pathway.

5.5A RIGHT ATRIAL PACING

In the presence of a left-sided accessory pathway, a right atrial impulse takes considerably longer to reach the pathway than it does to reach the AV node, and there may be minimal or no pre-excitation.

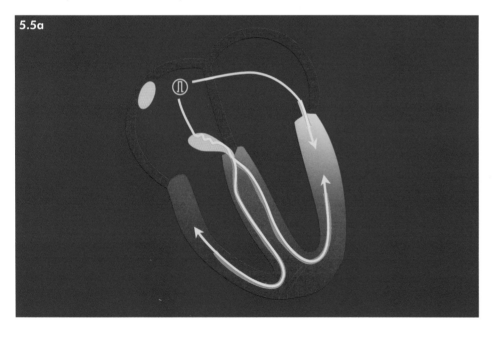

5.5a

5.5B CORONARY SINUS PACING

Pacing with an atrial catheter situated near the accessory pathway can make pre-excitation manifest. For left-sided pathways, this can be achieved by pacing in the CS. The atrial impulse reaches the pathway before the AV node, and the degree of pre-excitation is greatly increased.

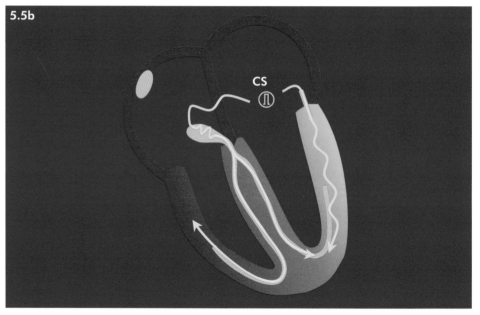

5.5b

CS

Differential atrial pacing can also be used to help locate accessory pathways. With left-sided pathways, the S-δ interval is shorter with pacing from the CS than that with pacing from the high right atrium. With right-sided pathways, pacing at various sites along the tricuspid annulus can be used to locate the site with the shortest S-δ interval.

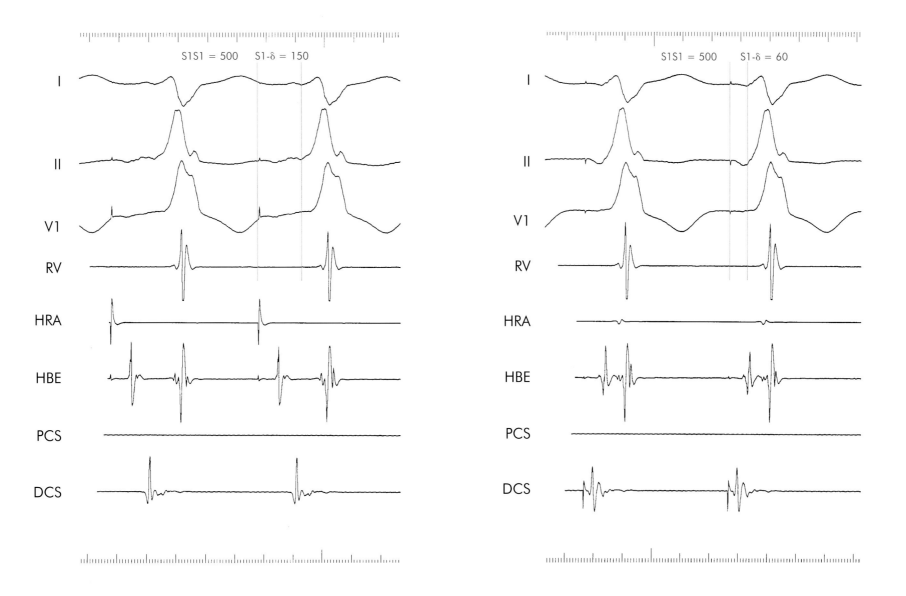

Tracing 5.5 Pacing is performed at a constant cycle length of 500 ms from the HRA (left panel) and the CS (right panel) in the same patient. CS pacing is associated with a shorter S-δ interval, indicating a left-sided accessory pathway. The S-δ interval is measured on the surface electrogram. There is no sensed intracardiac electrogram in the proximal coronary sinus (PCS) because that electrode pair is being used for pacing.

As with atrial pacing, pacing from different ventricular locations can be used to identify the presence and location of an accessory pathway during retrograde conduction.

5.6A RIGHT VENTRICLE APEX PACING

In the absence of an accessory pathway, atrial excitation can only occur over the AV node. A stimulus delivered at the right ventricle (RV) apex travels up the His-Purkinje system to the node.

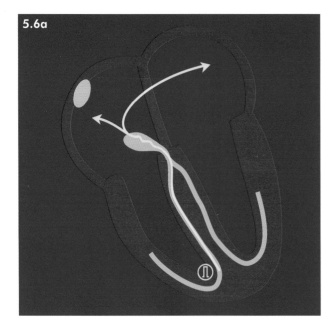

5.6B RV BASE PACING

A stimulus delivered at the RV base (or its outflow tract) has to reach the apex before invading the His-Purkinje system, and therefore takes longer to reach the atrium.

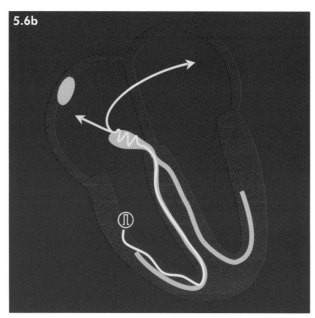

5.6C RIGHT-SIDED ACCESSORY PATHWAY

In the presence of a right-sided accessory pathway, the basal stimulus can reach the atrium more directly. The time taken to reach the atrium is the same or less (if the stimulus is near the pathway) than with RV apical pacing. This technique is particularly useful when the

earliest retrograde activation during RV pacing is at the CS os. Differential pacing can be used to distinguish between a posterior exit site for the AV node and a posteroseptal accessory pathway.

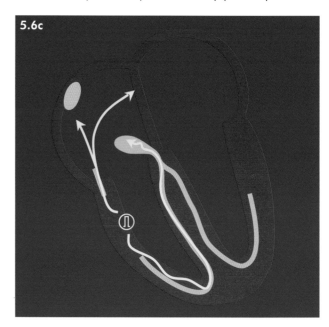

Similarly, left ventricular pacing can be used to accentuate atrial 'pre-excitation' by a left-sided accessory pathway. This can be useful to confirm the presence of a left-sided accessory pathway if there is difficulty in cannulating the CS.

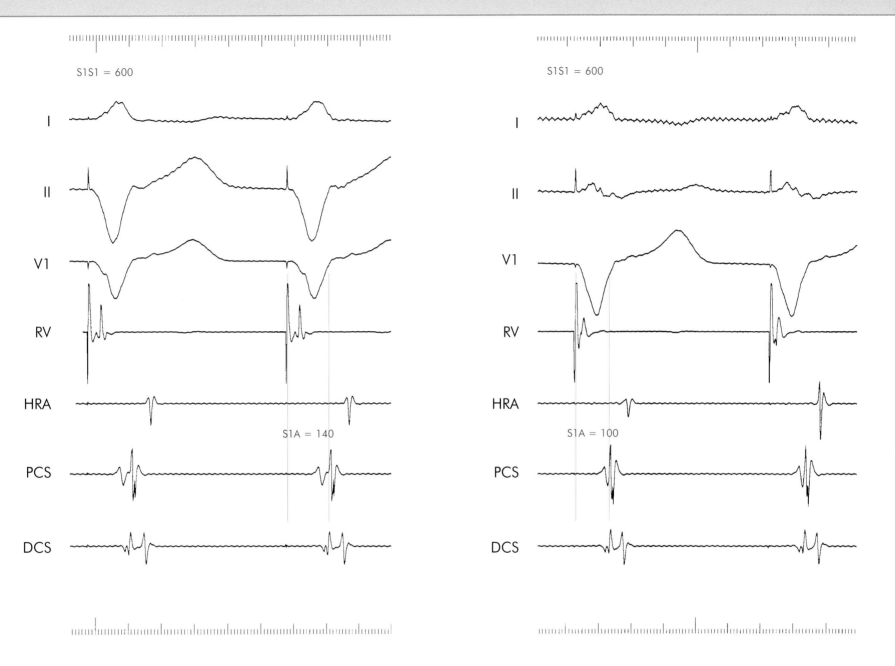

Tracing 5.6 Pacing from the right ventricular apex (left panel) demonstrates earliest activation at the proximal CS with a stimulus-to-atrial interval of 140 ms. After the catheter is positioned at the RV base (right panel; Figure 5.6c), the stimulus-to-atrial interval shortens to 100 ms, which is consistent with the diagnosis of a right posterior accessory pathway.

Retrograde conduction over a mid- or anteroseptal accessory pathway can be difficult to distinguish from conduction over the AV node as the pattern of atrial activation is concentric. Para-Hisian pacing can be used to identify the presence of an accessory pathway in this location. Pacing stimuli are delivered to the high RV septum just distal to the normal site for His bundle recording, adjacent to the His bundle and proximal right bundle branch. This is a special form of differential pacing in which variation of the pacing output, rather than the electrode location, is used to capture different structures selectively.

5.7A   NO PATHWAY — HIGH OUTPUT PACING

Pacing with a high output creates a strong enough current to capture the His bundle directly (Figure 5.7a). The impulse spreads directly to the AV node in the retrograde direction, and to the ventricles over the His-Purkinje system, giving a narrow QRS complex.

5.7B   NO PATHWAY — LOW OUTPUT PACING

The pacing output is reduced until direct capture of the His-Purkinje system no longer occurs and the ventricle is depolarized from the high septal myocardium (Figure 5.7b), leading to a left bundle branch block QRS morphology. The impulse has to travel to the apex to invade the His-Purkinje system retrogradely and, consequently, the time taken from the stimulus to atrial depolarization is greatly increased.

5.7C   ANTEROSEPTAL ACCESSORY PATHWAY

In the presence of an anteroseptal accessory pathway (AP) the atrium can be retrogradely activated from the high septum independently of the AV node. Thus, retrograde atrial activation is rapid whether the His-Purkinje system is directly stimulated (Figure 5.7c-i) or not (Figure 5.7c-ii).

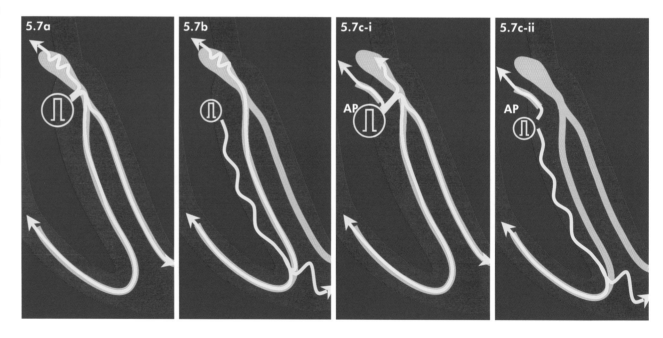

5.7a   5.7b   5.7c-i   5.7c-ii

Tracing 5.7 On beats two and three there is His capture: the surface QRS complex is narrow and the RV apex is activated early. On beats one and four there is loss of His capture: the surface QRS complex is wide and the time from stimulus to RV apex activation is long. There is very little prolongation of the VA interval with loss of His capture. This indicates that retrograde conduction is not solely over the node, and that an accessory pathway close to the anteroseptal region is probably present. In this example, the earliest activation is in the proximal CS throughout, and the accessory pathway was ablated in the midseptal region. In the absence of an accessory pathway, loss of His capture would be accompanied by prolongation of the VA interval by at least 50 ms.

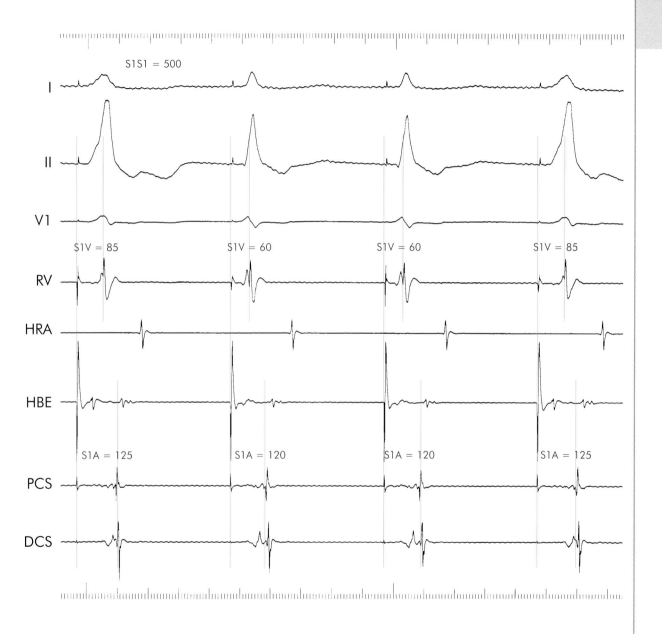

5.8A NOMENCLATURE OF ACCESSORY PATHWAY VARIANTS

Although the overwhelming majority of accessory pathways are atrioventricular (A), a number of unusual variants exist. Atriofascicular pathways (B) are the most frequent. Atrio-His pathways (C) bypass the AV node and terminate in the His bundle. Nodoventricular pathways (D) run from the AV node to the ventricular myocardium. Fasciculoventricular pathways (E), which are exceptionally rare, run from the bundle branches to the ventricular myocardium, activating part of the latter early.

5.8B RATE-DEPENDENT PATHWAYS

Some accessory pathways exhibit conduction properties similar to those of the AV node (slow, rate dependent, and often unidirectional). These are sometimes called 'decremental' pathways. Concealed (conducting V→A only) rate dependent atrioventricular pathways are fairly frequent. These are usually posteroseptal but occasionally seen in other locations, and are a cause of long RP' tachycardia (see Section 6.7).

Antegradely conducting rate dependent pathways are less common: the most frequent type is atriofascicular. These pathways usually originate at the anterolateral part of the tricuspid annulus and insert into the right bundle near the RV apex. Because of the slow conduction of the pathway, the surface ECG may show little or no pre-excitation during sinus rhythm. Pre-excitation can be made manifest with an atrial extrastimulus, especially if it is delivered near the origin of the pathway (Figure 5.8b). Because of the insertion of the pathway, the pre-excited QRS morphology usually resembles left bundle branch block (LBBB) with a left axis, and intracardiac recordings show earliest activation at the RV apex.

Antegradely conducting atrioventricular accessory pathways with rate-dependence are rare: these are again usually right-sided. Pre-excitation can be made manifest in the same way as with atriofascicular pathways, but as the insertion is at the AV annulus, the QRS morphology is less like LBBB with left axis deviation and depends on the pathway location. The RV apex is activated relatively late.

Connections causing ventricular pre-excitation with rate-dependence are often termed 'Mahaim fibers', but an anatomical description is now preferred to the loose use of an eponym. Mahaim originally ascribed the electrophysiological properties to a nodoventricular connection, but in the era of catheter ablation it has become clear that the cause is usually a pathway originating in the atrium, well away from the node (i.e. atriofascicular or atrioventricular).

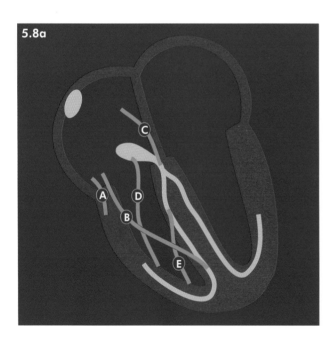

5.8a

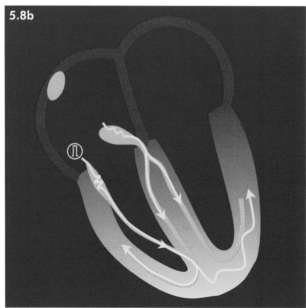

5.8b

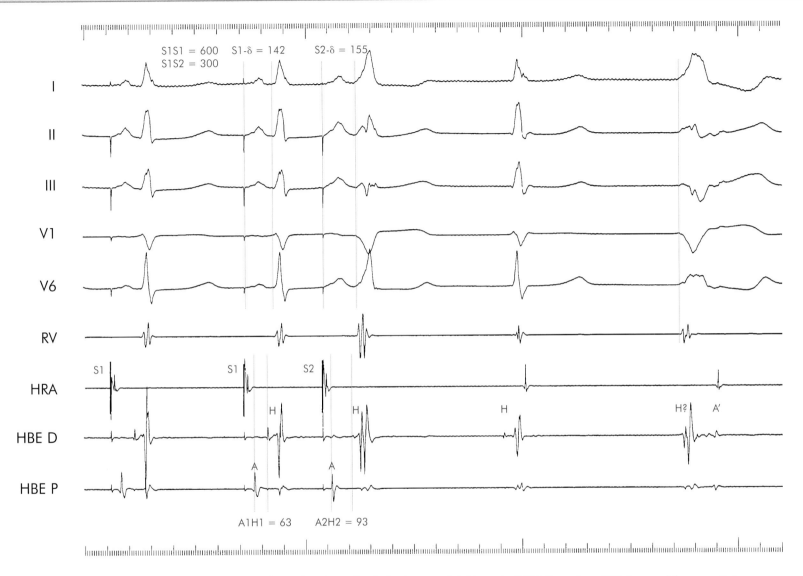

Tracing 5.8 This patient has a rate-dependent right-sided pathway (a form of 'Mahaim fiber'). During an atrial drive train (S1S1) the surface QRS shows subtle pre-excitation — compare leads II and III with the fourth beat in the tracing, which is a His extrasystole and therefore not pre-excited. Following an atrial extrastimulus (S2), the AH interval is prolonged due to delay in the AV node as usual. The S-δ interval is also slightly increased due to a slight delay in the pathway. However, this delay is less marked than that in the node, and as a result the QRS complex becomes more pre-excited.

The last beat in the tracing is an ectopic arising from the pathway itself, and conducted up the node to the atria (A', possibly preceded by a retrograde His potential). The fully pre-excited morphology of this beat has a horizontal rather than left axis, and the RV apical electrogram is ~20 ms after the onset of the QRS complex. These features suggest an atrioventricular rather than atriofascicular connection.

FURTHER READING

1. Anderson RH, Ho SY. Anatomy of the atrioventricular junctions with regard to ventricular preexcitation. Pacing Clin Electrophysiol 1997;20(8 Pt 2):2072–6.

2. Preexcitation syndromes. In: Prystowsky EN, Klein GJ. Cardiac Arrhythmias: An Integrated Approach for the Clinician. New York: McGraw-Hill, 1994:131–54.

3. Gallagher JJ, Pritchett EL, Sealy WC et al. The preexcitation syndromes. Prog Cardiovasc Dis 1978;20(4):285–327.

4. Miles WM, Zipes DP. Atrioventricular reentry and variants: mechanisms, clinical features and management. In: Zipes DP, Jalife J. Cardiac Electrophysiology: From Cell to Bedside. Philadelphia: WB Saunders, 1999:488–503.

5. Yee R, Klein GJ, Prystowsky E. The Wolff-Parkinson White Syndrome and related variants. In: Zipes DP, Jalife J. Cardiac Electrophysiology: From Cell to Bedside. Philadelphia: WB Saunders, 1999:845–61.

6. Fitzpatrick AP, Gonzales RP, Lesh MD et al. New algorithm for the localization of accessory atrioventricular connections using a baseline electrocardiogram. J Am Coll Cardiol 1994;23(1):107–16.

7. Hirao K, Otomo K, Wang X et al. Para-Hisian pacing. A new method for differentiating retrograde conduction over an accessory AV pathway from conduction over the AV node. Circulation 1996;94(5):1027–35.

8. Rosenthal LS, Calkins H. Catheter ablation of right freewall and Mahaim fibers. In: Singer I, editor. Interventional Electrophysiology. Baltimore: Williams and Wilkins, 1997:207–29.

9. Cosio FG, Anderson RH, Becker A et al. Living anatomy of the atrioventricular junctions. A guide to electrophysiological mapping. A Consensus Statement from the Cardiac Nomenclature Study Group, Working Group of Arrythmias, European Society of Cardiology, and the Task Force on Cardiac Nomenclature from NASPE. North American Society of Pacing and Electrophysiology. Eur Heart J 1999;20(15):1068–75.

10. Nodoventricular and facsiculoventricular bypass tracts. In: Josephson ME. Clinical Cardiac Electrophysiology, Second Edition. Philadelphia/London: Lea and Febiger, 1993:396–416.

Up to this point, we have discussed the substrates for supraventricular tachycardias (SVTs) and the methods used in the electrophysiology (EP) laboratory to demonstrate these. The next stage in diagnosis is the study of the tachycardia itself.

This section describes how information can be gleaned from observing the spontaneous and induced onset and termination of the tachycardia, as well as the effects of variation in the conduction of the components of the tachycardia circuit on the observed tachycardia. Methods used in the EP laboratory to distinguish tachycardia mechanisms using programmed atrial and ventricular stimulation will also be discussed. Finally, two important problems of differential diagnosis will be described — the so-called 'long RP' tachycardias' and pre-excited tachycardias.

The mode of onset of a tachycardia is often the most important clue to its mechanism.

6.1A ONSET OF AV NODAL REENTRANT TACHYCARDIA

The onset of atrioventricular nodal reentrant tachycardia (AVNRT) requires a critical prolongation in the AH interval, as the fast pathway blocks and conduction proceeds over the slow pathway (see Section 4.2).

6.1B ONSET OF AV REENTRANT TACHYCARDIA

AV reentrant tachycardia (AVRT) typically starts when a beat (sinus, ectopic or atrial extrastimulus) blocks in the accessory pathway, conducts to the ventricle over the AV node and can then return to the atria via the accessory pathway (see Section 5.4).

6.1C ONSET OF ATRIAL TACHYCARDIAS

The onset of atrial tachycardia may be accompanied by a degree of AH interval prolongation, but this is a secondary phenomenon, solely related to the increased atrial rate.

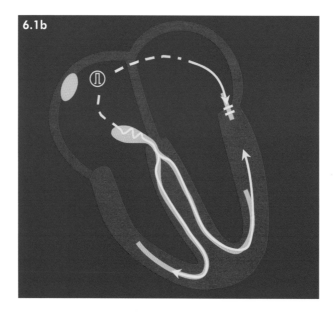

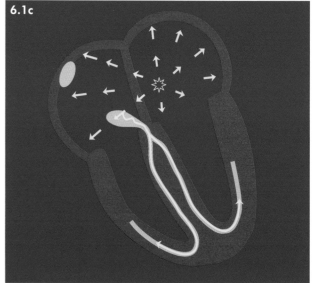

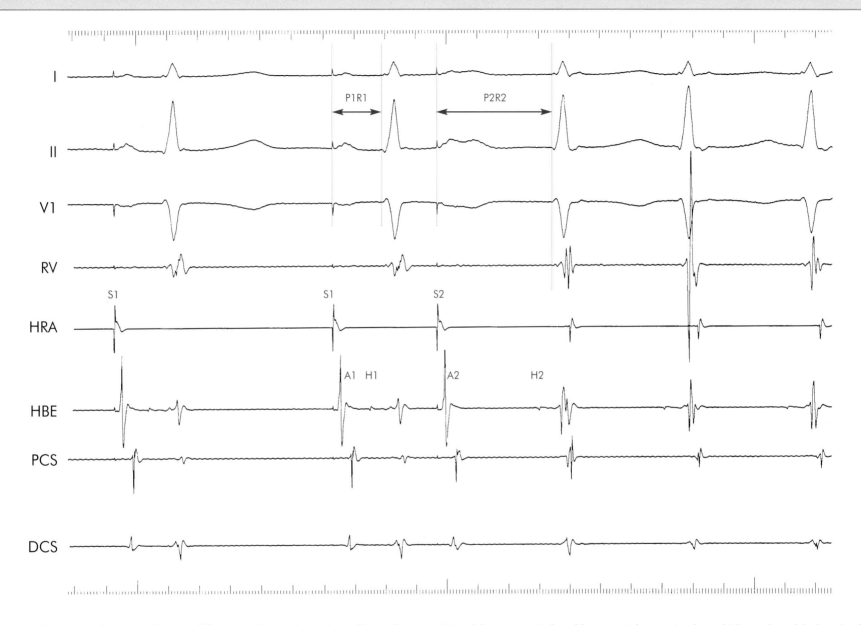

Tracing 6.1a The onset of tachycardia may differ according to the tachycardia mechanism. AV nodal reentry is induced by an atrial extrastimulus, which results in block in the fast pathway and conduction over the slow pathway. The AH prolongation is obvious but the mechanism can also be seen in the surface leads.

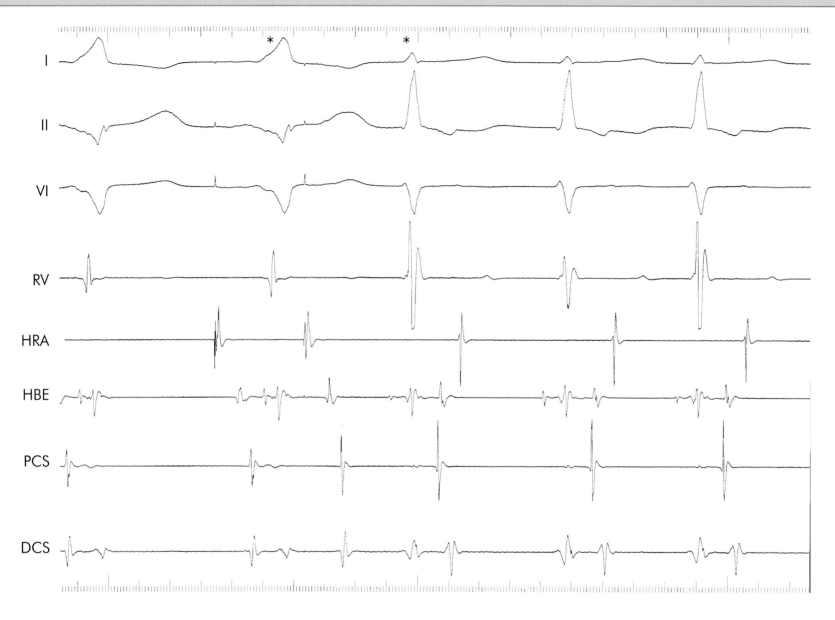

Tracing 6.1b Orthodromic AVRT is induced by an atrial extrastimulus. The key element of induction of tachycardia is block in the accessory pathway with loss of pre-excitation (*), allowing retrograde conduction up the accessory pathway to the atrium, thereby completing the circuit (see Section 5.4).

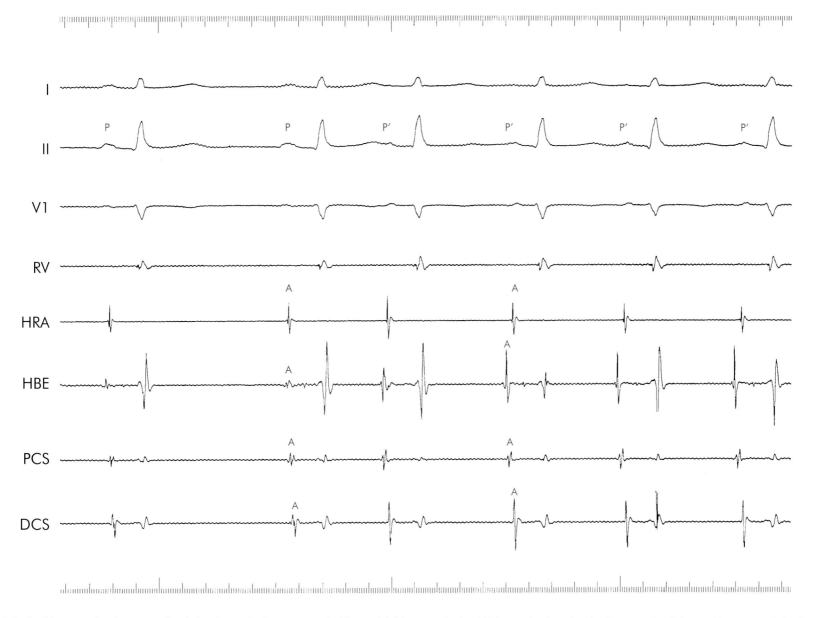

Tracing 6.1c In this example, the onset of atrial tachycardia is accompanied by a trivial increase in the AH interval, related to the increased atrial rate. However, subtle changes occur in the P-wave morphology between sinus rhythm (P) and tachycardia (P′), which correspond to slight changes in the atrial activation sequence seen on the intracardiac recordings. The observed AH interval makes AV reentry and AV node reentry very unlikely, since these are almost always associated with obvious AH prolongation.

Observing the termination of a tachycardia can also help distinguish between possible mechanisms. AV nodal-dependent tachycardias (AVNRT and AVRT) most commonly terminate when conduction is blocked in the AV node; this can be spontaneous or induced by drugs or vagal maneuvers.

6.2A COMMON TERMINATION OF AVNRT

Termination of AVNRT is usually due to block in the slow pathway. This means that for typical AVNRT (see Section 4) the atrial electrogram is usually the last visible event.

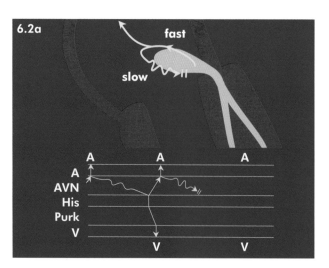

6.2B COMMON TERMINATION OF AVRT

The last visible event in termination of AVRT with block in the AV node is again an atrial electrogram.

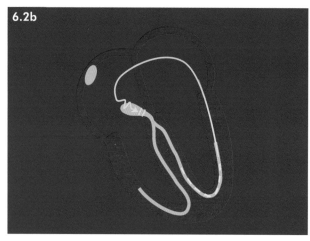

6.2C UNCOMMON TERMINATION OF AVRT AND AVNRT

Less commonly, the last event is a ventricular electrogram, due to block in the accessory pathway for AVRT (Figure 6.2c), or the retrograde AV nodal pathway for AVNRT.

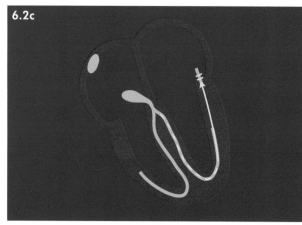

6.2D COMMON TERMINATION OF ATRIAL TACHYCARDIA

When atrial tachycardia with 1:1 AV conduction ceases, the last beat is usually conducted normally, so a ventricular electrogram is the last visible event. It is a rare coincidence for AV block to occur on exactly the same beat that the tachycardia itself terminates. Therefore, if the last visible event of the tachycardia is an atrial electrogram, atrial tachycardia is an unlikely diagnosis; if this is a consistent finding, the diagnosis can be virtually ruled out.

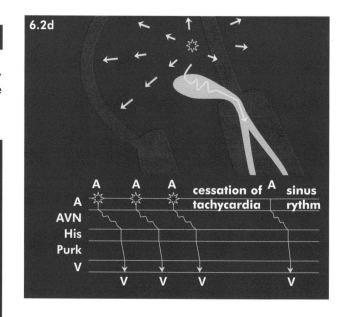

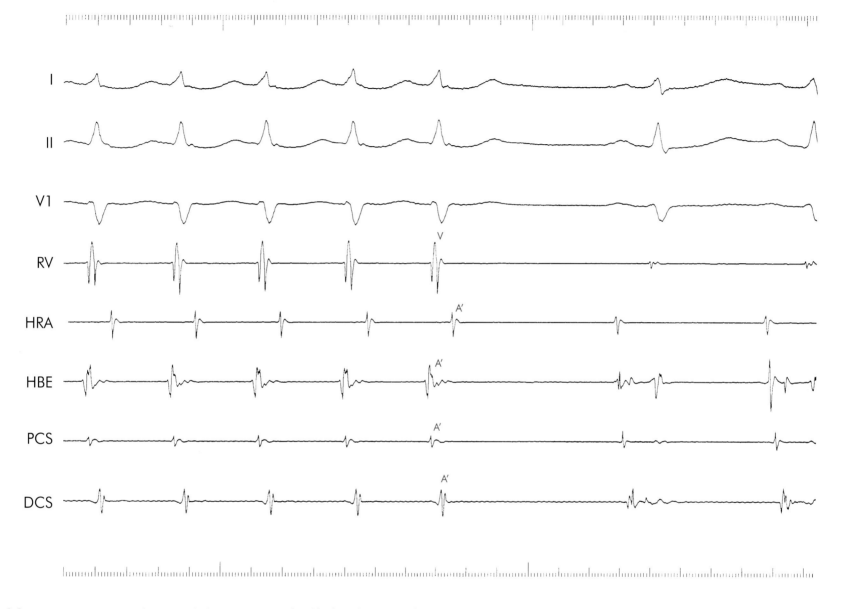

Tracing 6.2a AVNRT terminates with an atrial electrogram (A') after block in the slow pathway. Thus, the last event visible in AV nodal-dependent tachycardias (AVNRT and AVRT) is very frequently (but not always) an atrial electrogram.

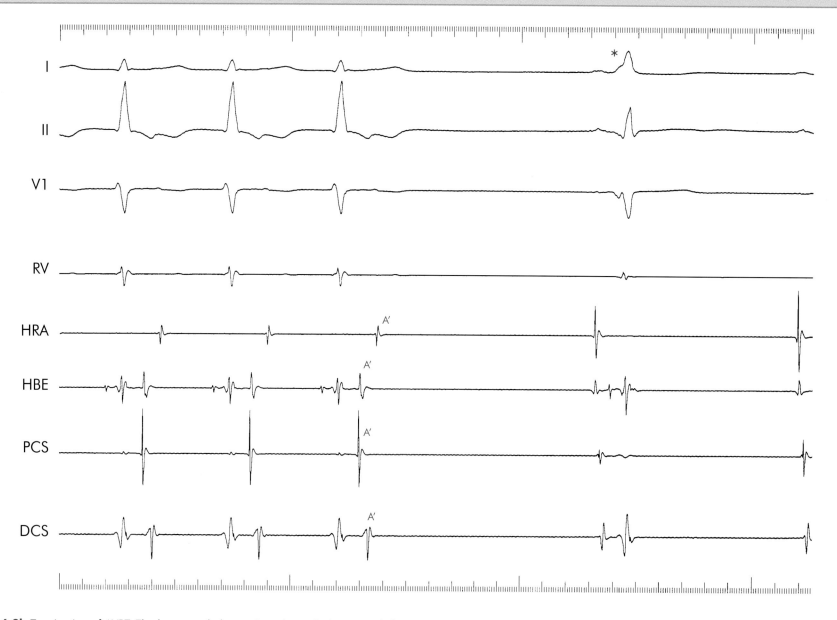

Tracing 6.2b Termination of AVRT. The last recorded event in tachycardia is an atrial electrogram (A'), indicating that tachycardia terminates with block in the AV node. The next beat is sinus rhythm with pre-excitation (*). This is the typical mode of termination for an AV node-dependent tachycardia, but unusual for an atrial tachycardia (see Section 6.2D).

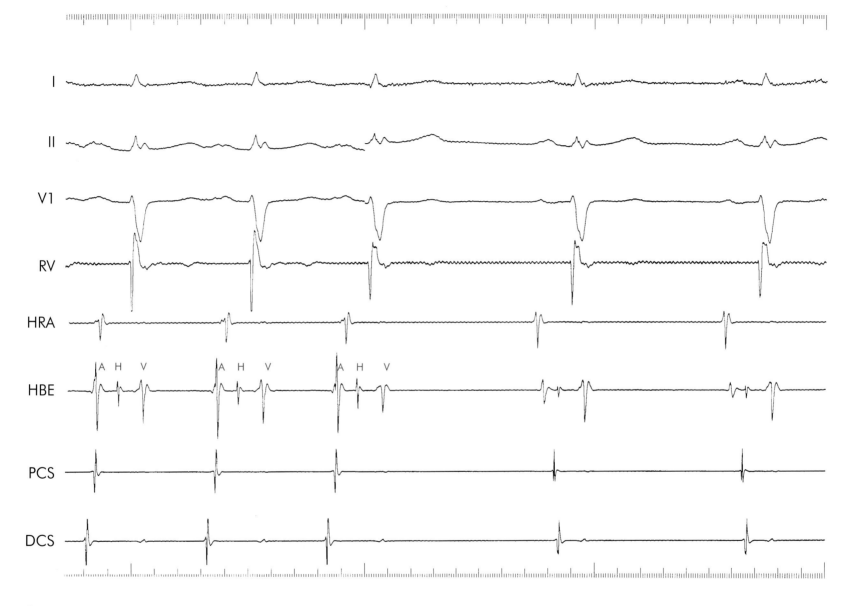

Tracing 6.2d Termination of a left atrial tachycardia. Note the change in surface P-wave accompanied by a complete change in the intracardiac atrial activation sequence. The last beat of the atrial tachycardia is conducted to the ventricles. Thus the last event is a ventricular electrogram, followed by resumption of sinus rhythm.

Minor cycle length irregularity is frequently seen, or can be induced by pacing, in SVTs.

In AVRT and typical AVNRT, any cycle length variation is usually caused by changes in the conduction time over the antegrade limb of the AV node, as this part of the circuit is highly dependent on cycle length and autonomic tone. Conversely, conduction over the His-Purkinje system to the ventricles, and over the accessory pathway or fast pathway back to the atria, tends to be very stable. Thus, the AH interval may vary but the HA' usually does not.[†]

The following rule is very useful: changes in the HH interval that precede and predict changes in the subsequent AA interval prove that the AV node participates in the reentrant circuit.

[†]The HA' may occasionally vary in the presence of His-Purkinje disease, which is usually obvious (e.g. bundle branch block), or accessory pathways with decremental retrograde conduction (see Section 6.7C).

6.3A CYCLE LENGTH VARIATION IN AVRT

Figure 6.3a shows AVRT with variation in the cycle length due to fluctuations in AV nodal conduction. The HA intervals are constant and each HH interval predicts the subsequent AA interval.

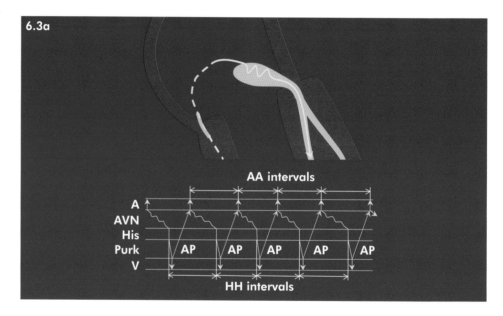

6.3a

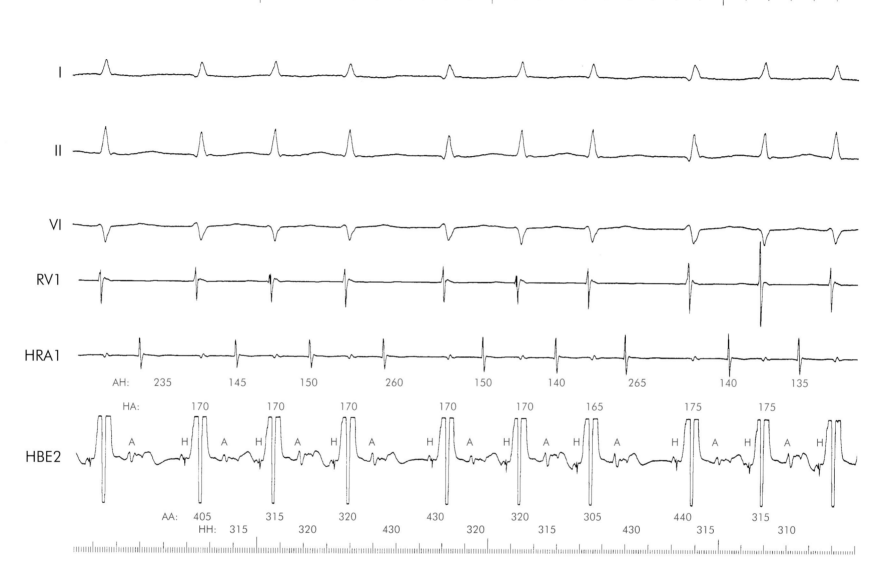

Tracing 6.3a Cycle length variation (obvious on the surface ECG) during AVRT. This variation is accounted for solely by changes in the AH interval, which probably represent shifts between conduction over the fast and slow AV nodal pathways. The HA interval is constant throughout, reflecting non-decremental conduction back to the atria via the ventricles and the accessory pathway. An irregular atrial tachycardia would give the appearance of variation in the HA interval. Another way of expressing this interpretation is that changes in the HH interval precede and predict changes in the AA interval, so this must be an AV node-dependent tachycardia.

6.3B   CYCLE LENGTH VARIATION IN ATRIAL TACHYCARDIA

Figure 6.3b shows atrial tachycardia with variable cycle length. The HH intervals do not predict the subsequent AA intervals as the principal variations are in the atrial tachycardia itself and these are independent of the AV node. Additionally, the AV node conduction may vary in response to changes in atrial cycle length, so the AA interval only approximately predicts the HH interval.

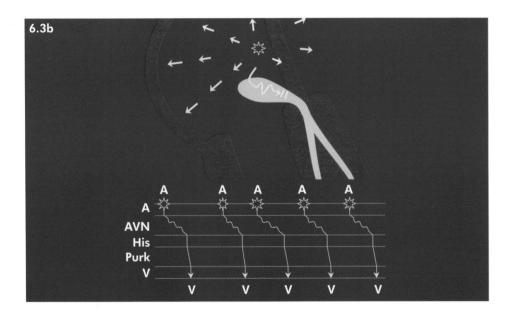

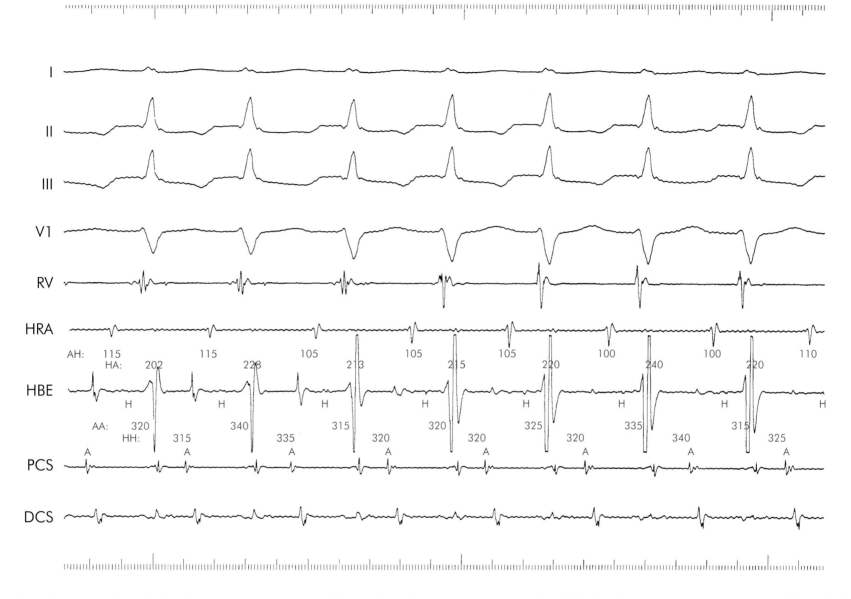

Tracing 6.3b Atrial tachycardia originating in the posteroseptal region of the low right atrium, near the coronary sinus (CS). The atrial electrogram in the proximal CS is earliest. The HA interval varies by up to 38 ms, and this is most compatible with an atrial tachycardia. The smaller variations in the AH interval reflect the normal response of the AV node to changes in cycle length. Another way of expressing the interpretation is that variations in the AA interval approximately predict the subsequent HH interval, but are not predicted by the preceding HH interval.

Atrioventricular (AV) dissociation is most commonly caused by AV block, which can be induced in the EP laboratory by: (1) vagal maneuvers; (2) the use of drugs such as adenosine and verapamil; or (3) making the AV node refractory with PACs or PVCs. The effects of AV dissociation can help distinguish between tachycardia mechanisms.

Atrial arrhythmias such as ectopic atrial tachycardia and atrial flutter are independent of AV nodal conduction, and can continue when AV block is induced.

6.4A AV BLOCK DURING ATRIAL TACHYCARDIA

Adenosine causes AV block during atrial tachycardia. Occasionally, it terminates the tachycardia but, even then, AV block is usually seen first, thereby establishing the diagnosis.

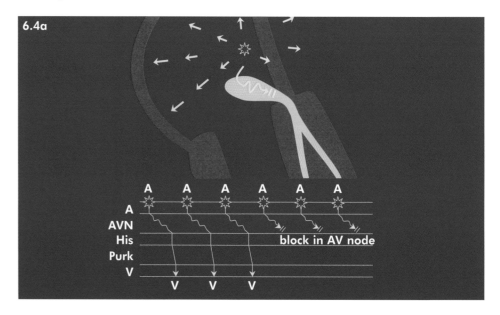

6.4a

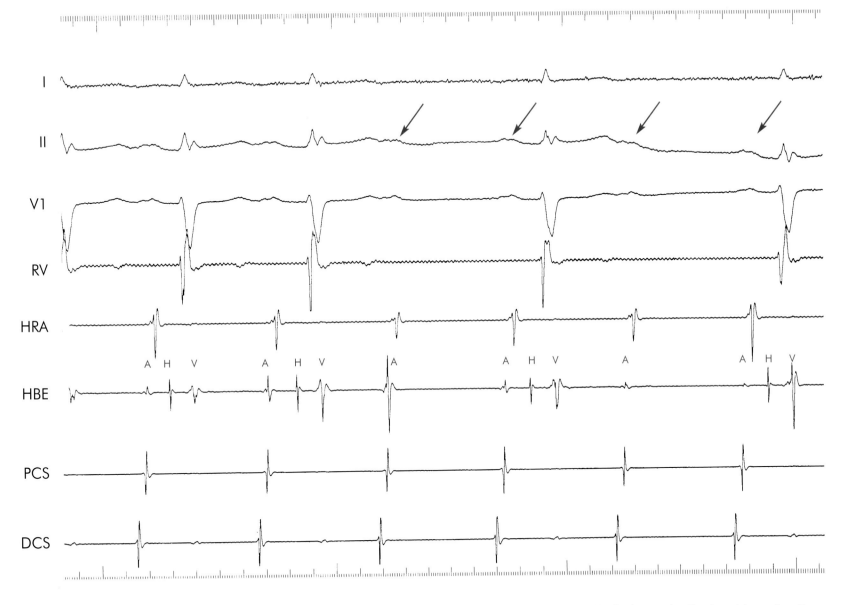

Tracing 6.4a Intravenous adenosine (6 mg) given during a left atrial tachycardia causes 2:1 block in the AV node. Adenosine also facilitates identification of the surface P-waves, which are best seen in lead II (arrowed).

6.4B   AV BLOCK IN AVNRT AND AVRT

The reentrant circuits of AVNRT and AVRT involve the AV node and are terminated by AV nodal block (induced, for example, by adenosine — see Section 5.2).

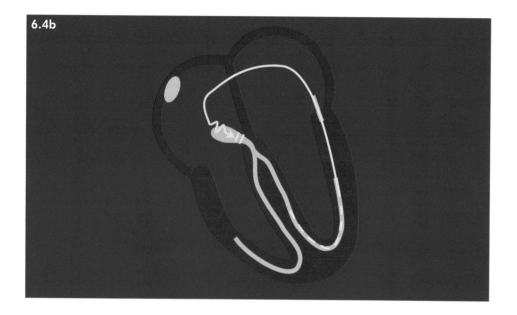

6.4b

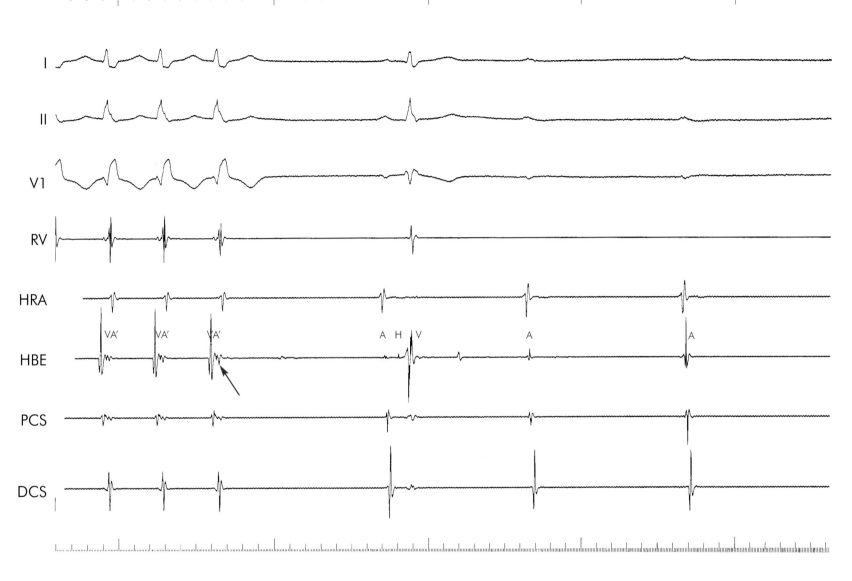

Tracing 6.4b Intravenous adenosine (6 mg) terminates AVNRT (with right bundle branch block) with an atrial electrogram (arrow). Sinus rhythm resumes with transient block in the AV node.

6.4C BLOCK BELOW THE NODE IN AVNRT

Atrial dissociation from the AVNRT circuit has been reported but is extremely rare. As a rule, if the atria can be dissociated from the tachycardia, the diagnosis is neither AVNRT nor AVRT.

AVNRT with spontaneous 2:1 conduction block below the node can, however, occasionally be seen — in this circumstance, there are more P-waves than QRS complexes. This can be suspected from the surface ECG when narrow P-waves with a low-to-high axis are seen midway between QRS complexes (alternating with P-waves that are buried in the QRS complexes). The P-wave morphology suggests that this is not simply typical atrial flutter with 2:1 conduction.

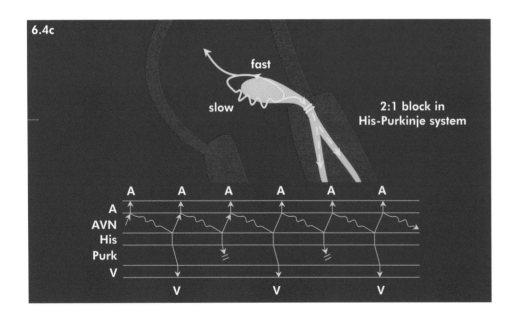

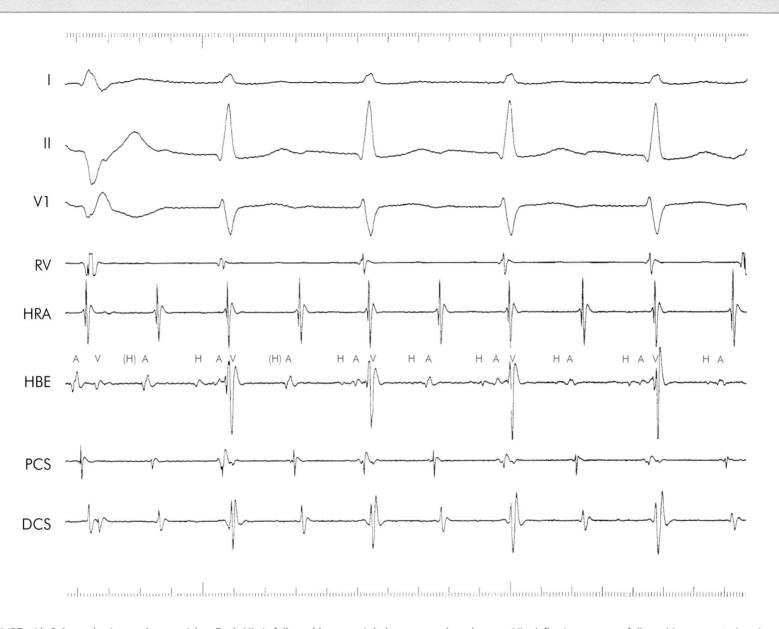

Tracing 6.4c AVNRT with 2:1 conduction to the ventricles. Each His is followed by an atrial electrogram, but alternate His deflections are not followed by a ventricular electrogram.

6.4D RAPID VENTRICULAR PACING IN AVNRT

AV dissociation can be induced by means other than AV block. During AVNRT, the ventricle can sometimes be paced faster than the tachycardia cycle length without interrupting the tachycardia. The ventricular impulses collide with those from the tachycardia below the AV node and the reentrant circuit is unaffected. This type of AV dissociation rules out ventricular participation in the tachycardia (i.e. AVRT) but is compatible with either an atrial tachycardia or AVNRT.

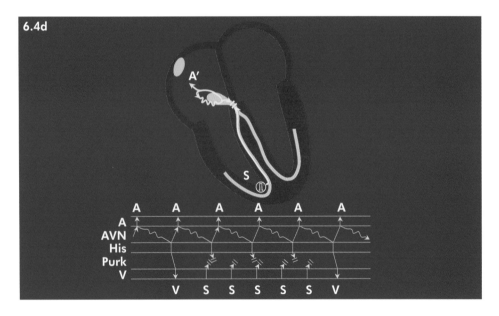

6.4E JUNCTIONAL ECTOPIC TACHYCARDIA

A special kind of tachycardia that does not appear to have a reentrant mechanism is junctional ectopic tachycardia (JET; also known as His bundle tachycardia), in which an automatic focus, presumably within the AV node, excites the His-Purkinje system from above. The appearance is of a narrow complex tachycardia that is unaffected by atrial or ventricular pacing. In contrast to AVNRT, this tachycardia may conduct intermittently to the atria or not at all. JET is classically seen in congenital heart disease, especially early after surgery. It is probably caused by injured AV nodal tissue that is potentiated by catecholamines. JET is rare in adults but a virtually identical appearance is characteristically seen during slow pathway ablation for AVNRT (see Section 8.3).

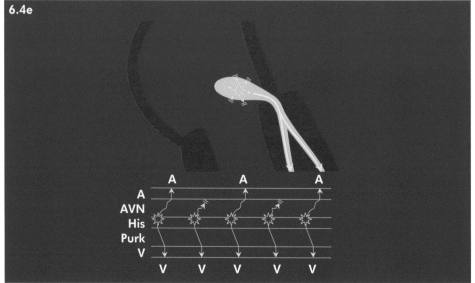

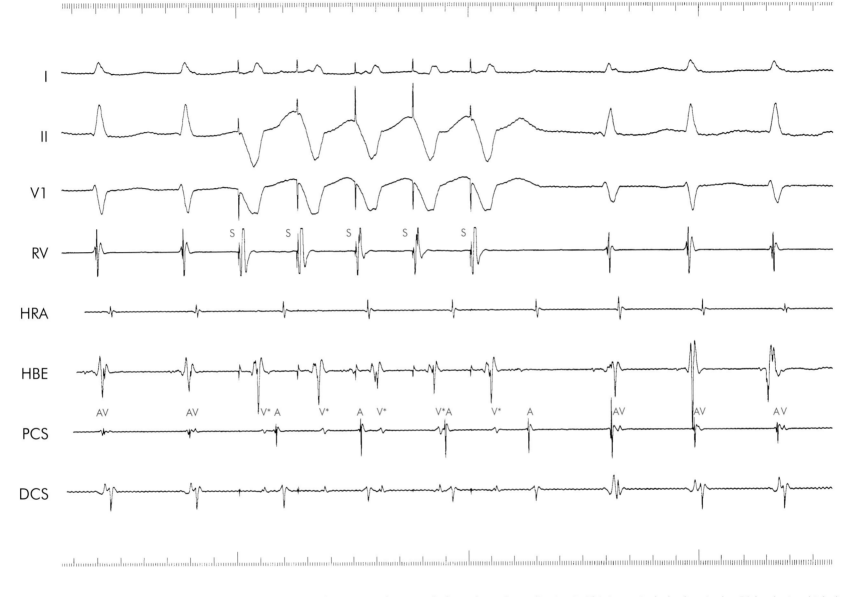

Tracing 6.4d A burst of ventricular pacing is delivered during AVNRT, dissociating the ventricle from the tachycardia circuit. This is particularly clear in the CS leads, in which the atrial activation is seen to be unaffected by the rapid ventricular impulses that result from pacing (V*).

If bundle branch block increases the cycle length of an SVT or the VA interval, the affected bundle branch must be part of the circuit.

6.5A ORTHODROMIC AVRT

Figure 6.5a shows an orthodromic AVRT, involving a left free wall accessory pathway. The circuit involves the left bundle branch.

6.5B EFFECT OF IPSILATERAL BUNDLE BRANCH BLOCK

In the presence of left bundle branch block (LBBB) the circuit can only return to the accessory pathway via the right bundle and slow conduction across the septum and through the left ventricular myocardium. The time taken to return to the atrium is increased (VA prolongation). If the bundle branch block persists, the tachycardia cycle length is also increased.

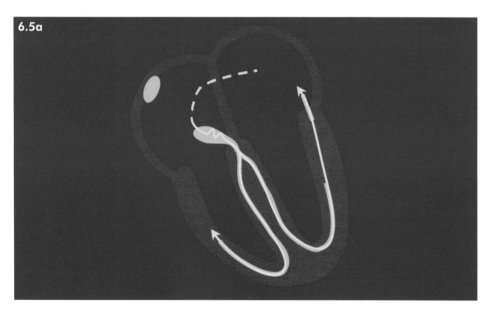

6.5a

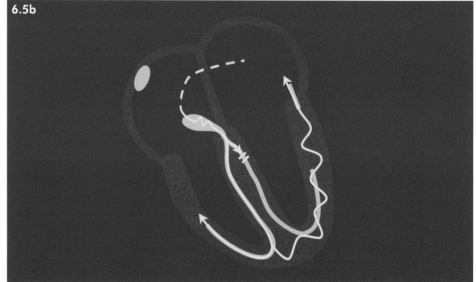

6.5b

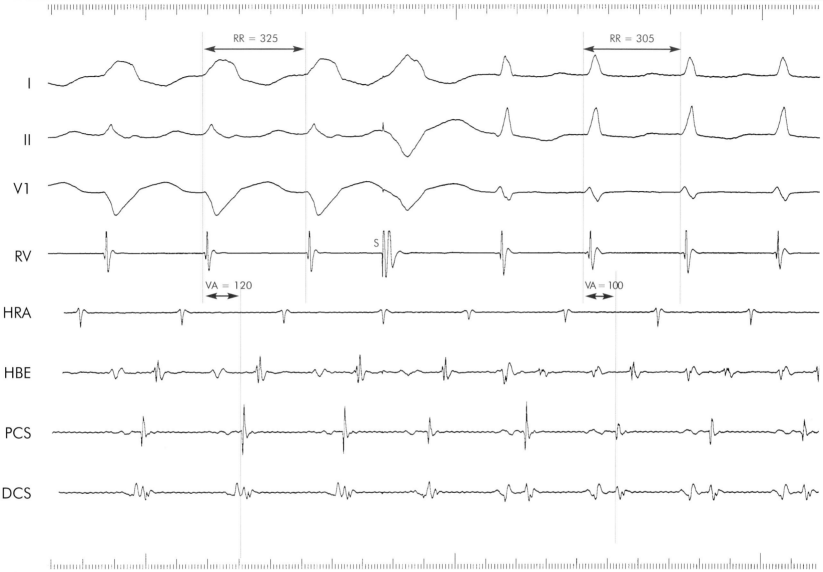

Tracing 6.5b AVRT with a left lateral accessory pathway. The first four beats show LBBB and the VA interval is 120 ms. Following a PVC (S), LBBB disappears and the VA interval shortens to 100 ms, with consequent shortening in the tachycardia cycle length. It is thus demonstrated that the left bundle branch participates in the circuit. Increase in tachycardia cycle length with bundle branch block is proof that the bundle, and by inference an ipsilateral accessory pathway, is part of the circuit.

Note that the ventricular signals in the coronary sinus electrogram give a misleading impression of the VA interval. During LBBB, these signals arrive late compared to global ventricular activation, so, although the true VA interval is long, the local VA is short. The converse occurs when LBBB ceases. This illustrates the importance of measuring the VA interval from the very earliest ventricular activation (here, as is usual, the beginning of the surface QRS complex).

6.5C CONTRALATERAL BUNDLE BRANCH BLOCK

RBBB will not affect a tachycardia involving a left free wall pathway. By the same token, AVRT involving a right-sided accessory pathway is only affected by RBBB. Ipsilateral bundle branch block may increase the VA interval (measured from the earliest ventricular signal to the earliest atrial signal) by 50 ms or more if a left or right free wall accessory pathway is involved. AVRT using an anteroseptal accessory pathway may show slight VA prolongation with RBBB but not LBBB, while the converse is seen in AVRT using a posteroseptal accessory pathway.

Thus, VA prolongation accompanying bundle branch block confirms the participation of an ipsilateral accessory pathway in the tachycardia circuit. The tachycardia cycle length is not always increased, however, as there may be a degree of compensation in the AV node, shortening the AH interval.

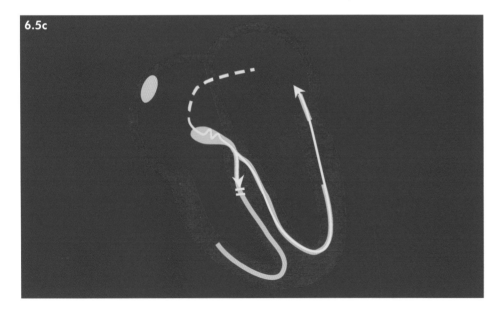

6.5c

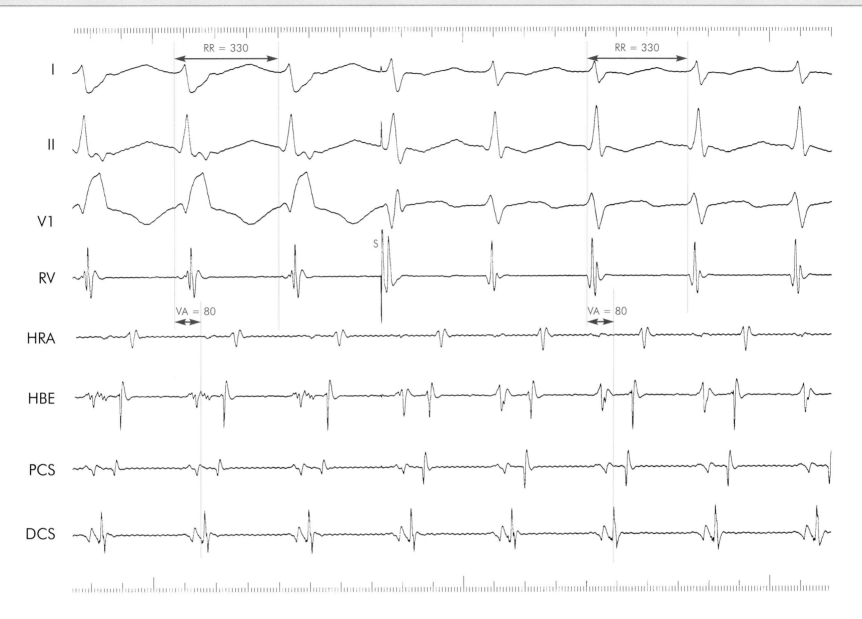

Tracing 6.5c AVRT with a left lateral accessory pathway. In the left half of the tracing, there is RBBB (most obvious in lead V1), which resolves with delivery of a single ventricular extrastimulus. This has no effect on the VA interval (and consequently none on the tachycardia cycle length), indicating that the right bundle branch (RBB) is not part of the circuit.

Critically timed premature ventricular contractions (PVCs) can help to determine the presence or absence of accessory AV pathways.

6.6A   PVC DELIVERY DURING AVRT

During AVRT the delivered PVC collides with and extinguishes the advancing tachycardia wavefront below the bundle of His. However, the PVC also propagates in the direction of the circuit, reaching the accessory pathway earlier than the tachycardia would have done. The next atrial activation is earlier than would be expected.

A PVC that is timed to coincide with the His bundle deflection (termed His-synchronous) cannot reach the atrium via the AV node as the His bundle is refractory. Atrial advancement by a His-synchronous PVC is therefore proof of the existence of another 'route' to the atria, i.e. an accessory pathway that conducts retrogradely.[†] However, it is not absolute proof that the pathway is part of the reentrant circuit — although rare, it is possible for a patient to have AVNRT and a 'bystander' accessory pathway.

If the atrium is advanced during AVRT by a PVC, there may be a degree of compensatory delay in the AV node (due to its decremental conduction) on the next beat. Thus, atrial advancement does not always lead to equal advancement of the whole circuit.

[†]This statement can probably be expanded to include PVCs introduced at the RV apex up to 50 ms either side of the anticipated His activation. Because of their timing, such signals cannot be conducted retrogradely over the His bundle.

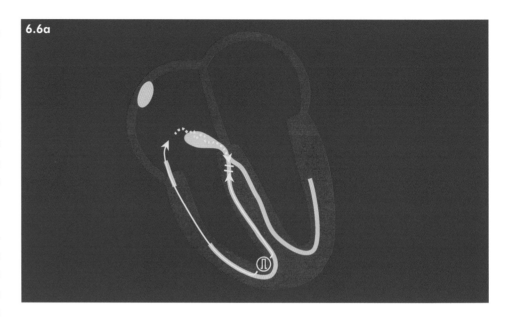

6.6a

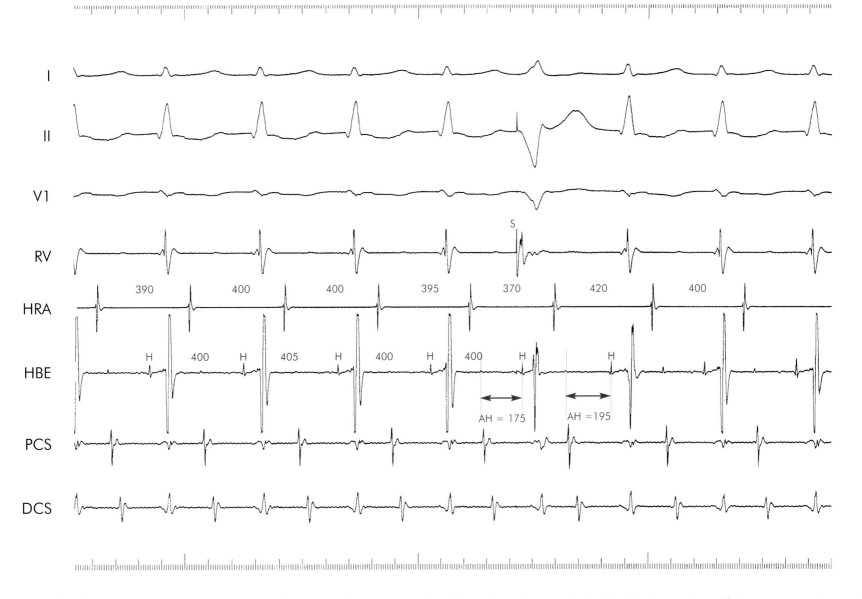

Tracing 6.6a AVRT with a right anterior accessory pathway. A single ventricular extrastimulus (S) is delivered just prior to the His deflection without affecting its timing. The result is advancement of the subsequent atrial electrogram by 30 ms, as measured in the high right atrium. An accessory pathway must therefore be present. Note that the tachycardia cycle length is very stable prior to the PVC; if there were significant 'wobble', it would be difficult to be certain that the advanced atrial electrogram was indeed due to the PVC. The early atrial activation results in an increased AH interval. As a result the whole circuit is only marginally advanced.

6.6B TACHYCARDIA TERMINATION BY HIS-SYNCHRONOUS PVC

A PVC delivered when the His bundle is refractory may reach the accessory pathway when it is also refractory. The PVC is therefore not conducted to the AV node or the atrium. SVT termination by a His-synchronous PVC that does not reach the atria is proof of the participation of the ventricle, and therefore an accessory pathway, in the circuit.

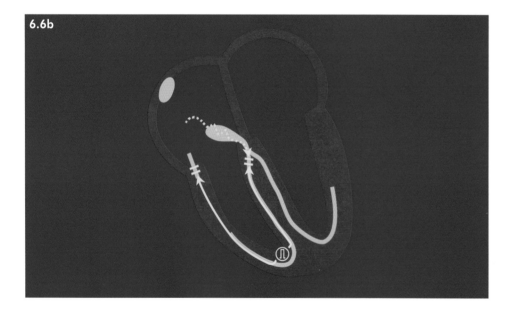

6.6b

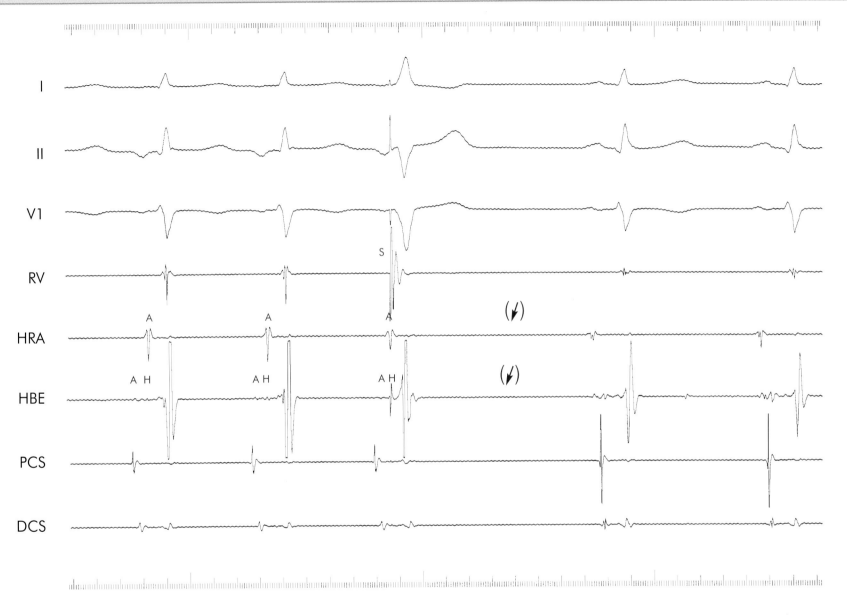

Tracing 6.6b An unusual form of AVRT using a slowly conducting posteroseptal accessory pathway (a cause of long RP' tachycardia — see Section 6.7). A single ventricular extrastimulus (S), timed to coincide with His activation, terminates the tachycardia without conduction to the atrium (no atrial electrogram where expected, at arrow), proving that the ventricle (and thus an accessory pathway) is a necessary part of the circuit.

6.6C   PRE-EXCITATION INDEX

A PVC may not succeed in penetrating the reentrant circuit and pre-exciting the atrium if it is delivered remote from the circuit. For example, a PVC delivered at the right ventricular apex may take 50 ms to cross the septum and reach a circuit involving a left-sided accessory pathway. To pre-excite the atrium in this case, it may be necessary to deliver the PVC nearer the circuit (e.g. in the left ventricle), or earlier than the His bundle timing (as shown in Figure 6.6c).

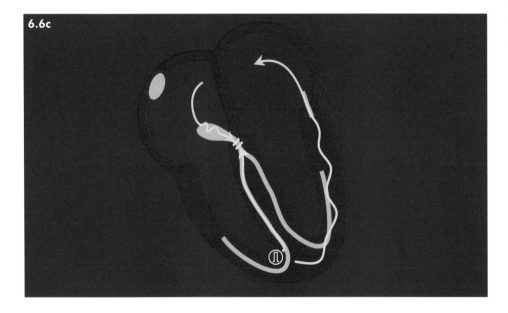

6.6c

The 'pre-excitation index' (PEI) is a tool that can help localize an accessory pathway based on this observation. Essentially it quantifies the concept that the further an accessory pathway is from the stimulation site, the greater the prematurity required for a PVC to reach that pathway. The PEI is defined as the prematurity of the latest right ventricle (RV) apical PVC that is able to advance the atrium. This prematurity is calculated as the tachycardia cycle length minus the coupling interval of the PVC. Using RV pacing, a PEI >75 ms suggests a tachycardia involving a left free wall pathway; a PEI <45 ms suggests a septal accessory pathway while intermediate values would be typical of a right free wall pathway. Very early PVCs (PEI >120 ms) can advance the atrium even in AVNRT, as with this degree of prematurity the His and retrograde fast pathway are often fully excitable.

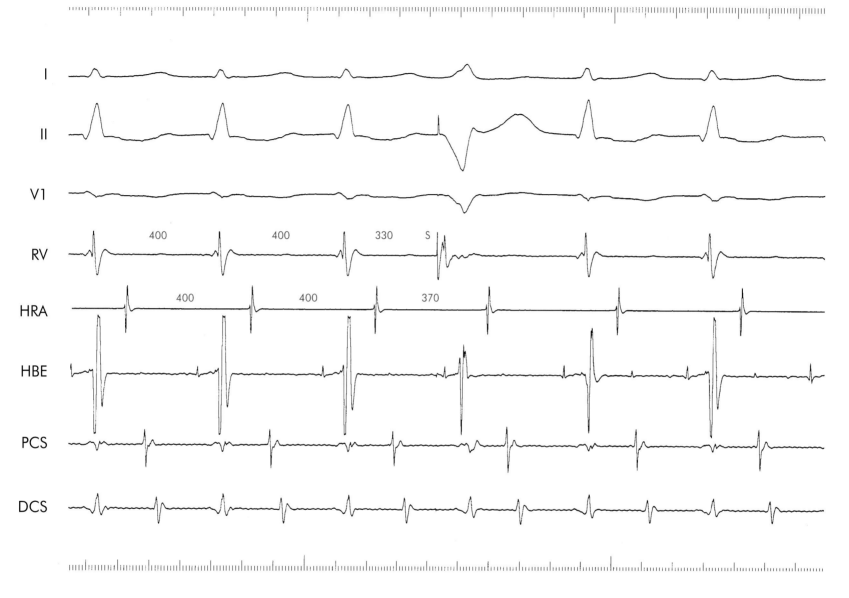

Tracing 6.6c AVRT with a right anterior accessory pathway. A single ventricular extrastimulus (S) is delivered just prior to the His deflection, whose timing it does not affect. The tachycardia cycle length is 400 ms. The PVC illustrated is the latest coupled PVC to advance the subsequent atrial electrogram as measured in the HRA. The VV interval of the PVC is 330 ms, 70 ms earlier than the expected tachycardia ventricular electrogram. Thus the PEI is 70 ms.

A regular narrow complex tachycardia in which the PR interval is shorter than the RP' interval is termed a 'long RP' tachycardia'. This can be due to: (i) atrial tachycardia; (ii) atypical AV node reentry of the 'fast-slow' variety (see Section 4.5C); or (iii) AVRT using a pathway that conducts slowly in the retrograde direction. Often, the pattern of tachycardia onset and/or the P-wave axis (e.g. sinus tachycardia) helps establish the mechanism. However, the differential diagnosis is less straightforward when atrial activation appears to arise from the low right atrium, as is commonly the case.

6.7A   LOW RIGHT ATRIAL TACHYCARDIA

The low right atrium, near the CS os, is a common location for an ectopic focus. For an example, see Tracing 6.3b (note the inverted P-wave in lead II).

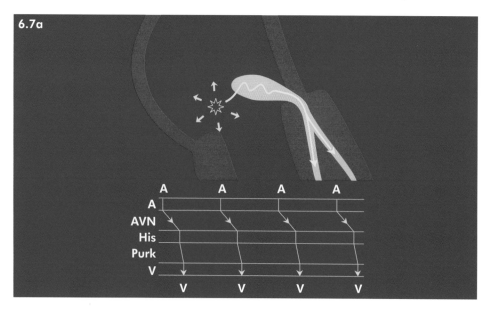

6.7B   ATYPICAL AVNRT — 'FAST-SLOW' VARIETY

The retrograde slow limb of the AVNRT circuit usually has its exit site in the low posterior septum, again near the CS os (see Section 4.5C).

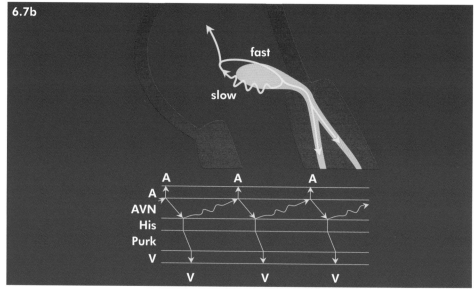

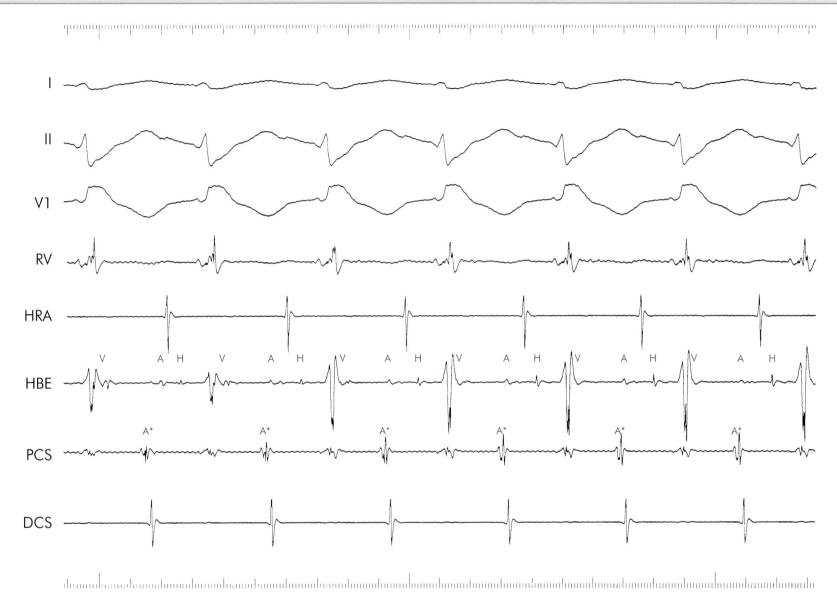

Tracing 6.7b Atypical AVNRT that uses a fast pathway antegrade and slow pathway retrograde. Because the slow pathway is posterior, the earliest atrial activation is seen at the CS os (A*). The long RP′ and short PR would be even more pronounced were it not for a long HV interval, indicating delay in the His-Purkinje system (note there is also RBBB).

6.7C   AVRT USING A DECREMENTAL POSTEROSEPTAL PATHWAY

The accessory pathway has a posteroseptal location and its retrograde conduction is decremental (and therefore slow during tachycardia). This tachycardia is classically seen in children and adolescents, is often incessant[†] over a period of months or years, and can eventually cause heart failure. It is also known as permanent junctional reciprocating tachycardia (PJRT).

It should be said that, while rate-dependent accessory pathways that only conduct in the retrograde direction are typically posteroseptal, they can occur in other locations, clues to which can come from the P-wave axis during tachycardia.

[†]Long RP' tachycardias are frequently 'incessant'. This term, which has a special meaning to electrophysiologists, is something of a misnomer. It does not refer to a tachycardia that never ceases, but rather to one that constantly restarts shortly after terminating. Such patients spend very little time in sinus rhythm, so it is often not possible to conduct a formal EP study of the arrhythmia substrate. The differential diagnosis is therefore based on the methods described earlier in this section (including observation of onset, termination, cycle length variation and effects of ventricular pacing).

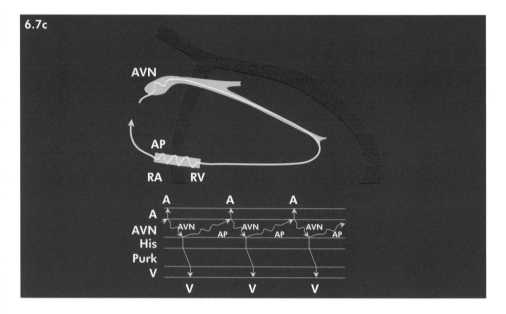

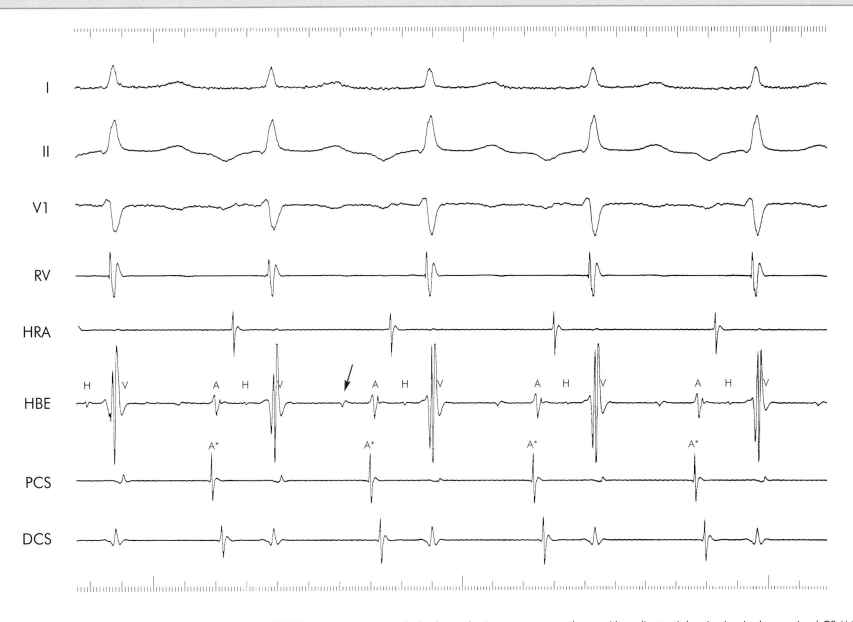

Tracing 6.7c Permanent junctional reciprocating tachycardia (PJRT) using a decremental, slowly conducting accessory pathway with earliest atrial activation in the proximal CS (A*). It is typical for this tachycardia that the surface P-waves are clear and have an upward axis. The small, sharp deflections (arrowed) are repolarization artifacts, which can sometimes cause confusion. In this patient they coincided with the T-wave in sinus rhythm as well as in tachycardia. The effects of PVCs during tachycardia (see Section 6.6) are critical to the distinction between AVNRT and AVRT in an example such as this.

Several tachycardias exist in which the ventricles are partly or solely activated by an accessory pathway. These are known as pre-excited tachycardias, and can be divided into two groups: (i) those in which pre-excitation is a passive (bystander) phenomenon, incidental to the tachycardia mechanism; and (ii) those in which the accessory pathway is an obligatory part of the tachycardia mechanism.

6.8A   PRE-EXCITED ATRIAL FIBRILLATION

Bystander pre-excitation can accompany any supraventricular tachycardia, the most common example being pre-excited atrial fibrillation (AF). Patients with accessory pathways are at increased risk of developing AF, possibly because of the effects of repeated episodes of AVRT on the electrophysiological properties of the atria. Figure 6.8a: as in sinus rhythm, the ventricles can be depolarized mostly over the accessory pathway (left), over the AV node (right), or by a fusion of both. A particularly common pattern is one of runs of QRS complexes with little or no pre-excitation alternating with runs of more fully pre-excited complexes.

If the accessory pathway has a short functional refractory period, it may give rise to shorter RR intervals during AF than would be allowed by conduction solely over the AV node. In exceptional circumstances, the ventricular response can be rapid enough to degenerate into ventricular fibrillation. This is thought to be the basis for the very small risk of sudden death in patients with the Wolff–Parkinson–White syndrome. The highest risk patients are those in whom the shortest RR interval during AF is <200 ms, or those in whom the accessory pathway effective refractory period (ERP) is <250 ms. Before catheter ablation became widespread, these parameters were measured at EP study, and intervention such as drug therapy or surgery was recommended for high-risk patients.

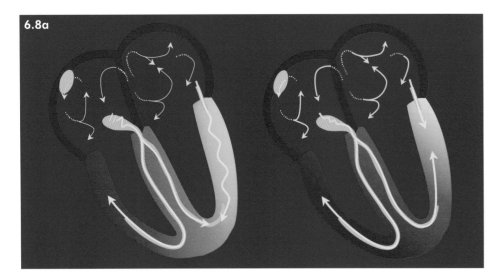

6.8a

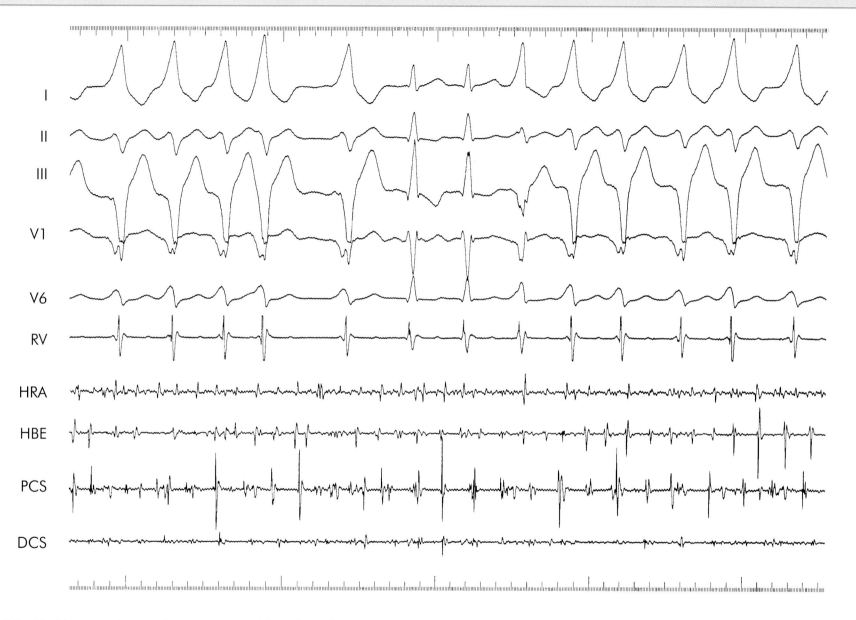

Tracing 6.8a AF with varying degrees of pre-excitation visible on the surface ECG. Note the rapid, irregular, low amplitude activity in the atrial electrograms characteristic of AF. The shortest RR interval in this segment of recording is around 250 ms, but elsewhere the patient exhibited intervals below 200 ms, indicating a potentially dangerous accessory pathway.

6.8B OTHER TACHYCARDIAS WITH BYSTANDER PRE-EXCITATION

Other tachycardias, such as atrial tachycardia (Figure 6.8b, left), atrial flutter and AVNRT (Figure 6.8b, right), can also be passively pre-excited by an accessory pathway. The result is a regular wide complex tachycardia that may resemble ventricular tachycardia (VT) on the surface ECG. A clue to the diagnosis may come from similarity between the pre-excited QRS morphology in sinus rhythm and tachycardia. To exclude VT formally it may be necessary to use techniques such as those in Section 6.4 to demonstrate that the ventricles can be dissociated from the tachycardia.

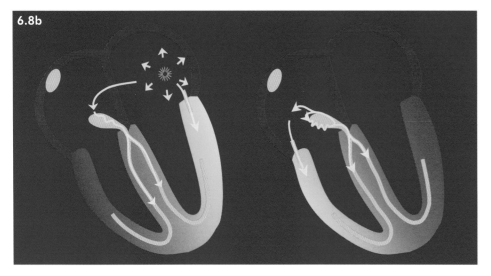

6.8b

6.8C ANTIDROMIC AVRT

In two forms of pre-excited tachycardia, conduction over the accessory pathway is obligatory. These are antidromic AVRT and pathway-to-pathway tachycardia.

In antidromic AVRT (Figure 6.8c, left), the usual AV reentrant circuit is reversed, with the impulse traveling down the accessory pathway and returning to the atria retrogradely over the His-Purkinje system and AV node. In this uncommon form of AVRT, the entire ventricle is activated over the accessory pathway (fully pre-excited). Note that the terms 'orthodromic' and 'antidromic' are used to describe tachycardias with His bundle participation in the normal (A→V) and reverse (V→A) directions, respectively.

Antidromic AVRT frequently uses a rate-dependent atriofascicular pathway (see Section 5.8). As these pathways usually insert into the distal His-Purkinje system near the right ventricular apex (Figure 6.8c, right), the QRS complex during tachycardia typically has an LBBB morphology with a leftward axis.

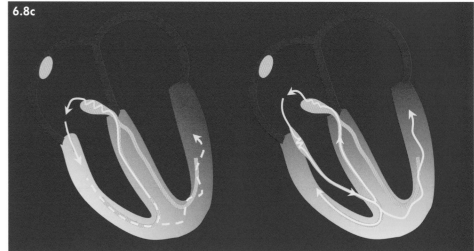

6.8c

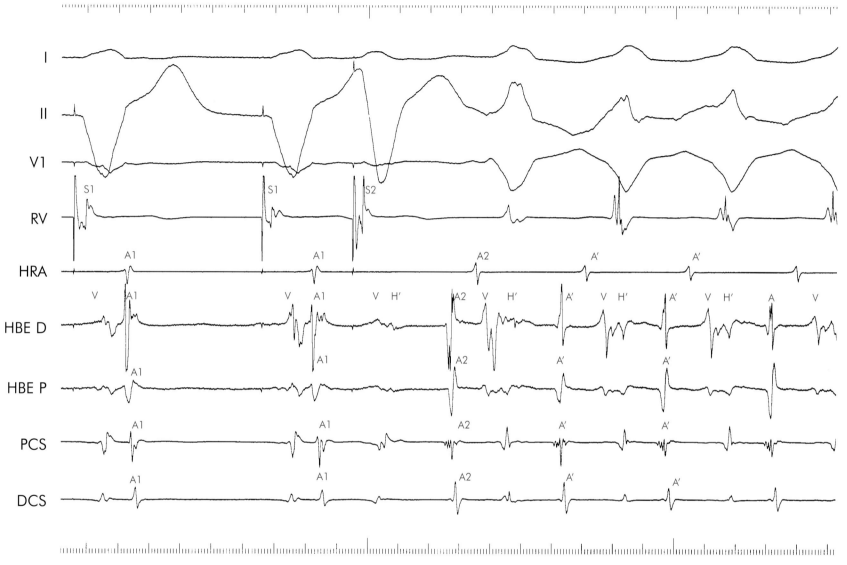

Tracing 6.8c Ventricular extrastimulus testing in a patient with a right anterior accessory atrioventricular pathway induces antidromic AVRT. During the drive train, earliest atrial activation is recorded simultaneously at the His and high right atrium (A1). This is abnormal and indicates retrograde conduction over an accessory pathway (see Section 5.3). With the extrastimulus, there is block in the accessory pathway and slow retrograde conduction over the AV node to the atrium, which is now concentrically activated (A2). The accessory pathway then conducts the impulse down to the ventricle, completing the circuit. Note that, during tachycardia, there is a retrograde His deflection (H'). This is followed (after a pause for retrograde AV nodal conduction) by concentric atrial activation, seen earliest in the His and proximal CS catheters (A'). Note also that the RV apex is activated late in relation to the QRS complex. As ventricular activation is entirely over the pathway, the surface QRS has a fully pre-excited appearance.

6.8D   DIAGNOSIS OF ANTIDROMIC AVRT

For antidromic AVRT to occur, the accessory pathway must be able to conduct antegradely. Ventricular pre-excitation is usually easy to demonstrate during the baseline EP study. The diagnosis of antidromic AVRT itself is based on the following findings:

• Fully pre-excited QRS morphology.

• Atrial activation is concentric (i.e. earliest atrial activity is recorded in the region of the AV node).

• Ventricular activation can be advanced by premature atrial contractions (PACs) without the involvement of the AV node — this is the counterpart of the method described in Section 6.6, in which PVCs are used to advance the atrium during orthodromic AVRT. To demonstrate this, it may be necessary to pace near the atrial insertion of the accessory pathway (Figure 6.8d). If the PAC advances the ventricle more than it advances the His potential or the atrium near the node, then it can only have done so over an accessory pathway (as in Tracing 6.8d-i). Similarly, if the PAC is simultaneous with atrial activation near the node yet advances the ventricle, it can only have done so over an accessory pathway (as in Tracing 6.8d-ii).

• Demonstration of retrograde activation of the His-Purkinje system. This can often be achieved using a closely spaced multipolar catheter to record His and right bundle branch potentials; in antidromic tachycardia, activation of the right bundle and distal His precedes that of the proximal His.

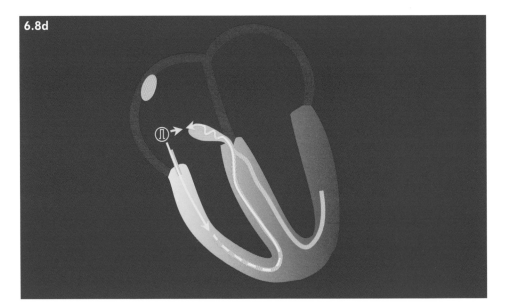

6.8d

150

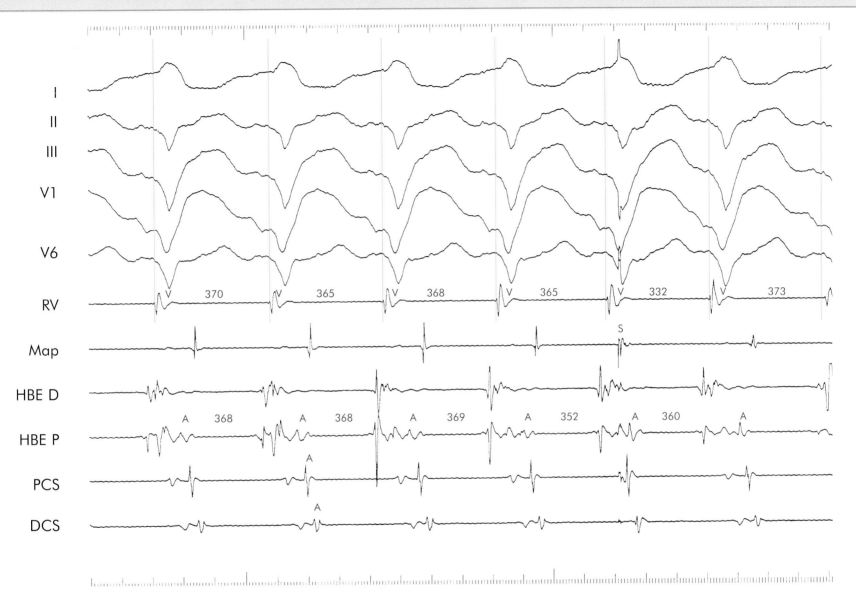

Tracing 6.8d-i Antidromic AV reentrant tachycardia using a right-sided atrioventricular accessory pathway. The tachycardia is fully pre-excited and atrial activation is concentric, suggesting that antegrade conduction is over an accessory pathway and retrograde conduction is over the AV node. The His spike is invisible, buried within the ventricular electrogram. A PAC is delivered by a steerable catheter (Map) approximately at a time when the next His might be expected. The extrastimulus advances the atrial electrogram near the node by 17 ms, but the next ventricular cycle is advanced by >30 ms. This can only have been by ventricular activation over an accessory pathway.

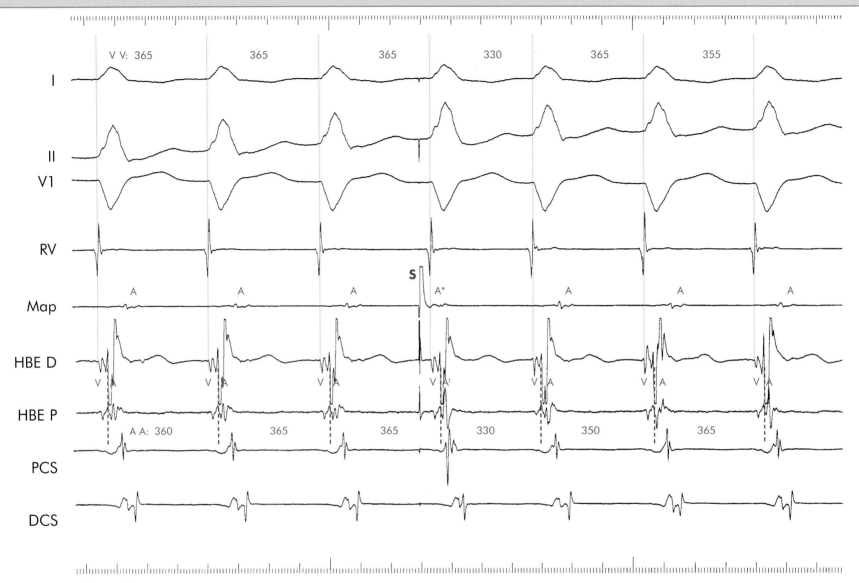

Tracing 6.8d-ii Antidromic AV reentrant tachycardia using an atriofascicular accessory pathway as its antegrade limb. As in Tracing 6.8d-i, the QRS is fully pre-excited and atrial activation is concentric. This mechanism can be confirmed by observing the response to an extrastimulus delivered in the right atrial free wall, near the pathway (S, A*). The extrastimulus advances the ventricle on the next beat and resets the tachycardia. The ventricle cannot have been advanced via the AV node as the atrium near the AV node, recorded in the His channel (A†), was unaffected by the PAC, and advancement must therefore have been over an accessory pathway. Note that the AV interval is long, and that, although the extrastimulus is 70 ms premature, the ventricular advancement is by only 35 ms. This is due to the slow, rate-dependent properties characteristic of this type of pathway. Note also that, because of the ventricular insertion into the distal right bundle, the RV apical electrogram is very early in relation to the surface QRS complex.

6.8E 'PATHWAY-TO-PATHWAY' TACHYCARDIA

In this tachycardia, activation travels from atrium to ventricle via one accessory pathway and returns via another. The AV node does not take an active part but may be passively activated in either direction. For this extremely rare tachycardia to be possible, the cycle length must be sufficiently slow to allow the tissue at each stage to recover from refractoriness. This means either that the two pathways are located distant from each other, or that at least one pathway is rate-dependent, conducting slowly during tachycardia. According to the definitions given earlier, this type of pre-excited tachycardia is neither truly orthodromic nor antidromic, as the AV node does not participate actively in the circuit. Keys to recognition of pathway-to-pathway tachycardia are: (i) that both atrium and ventricle are obligatory parts of the circuit; and (ii) atrial activation is eccentric.

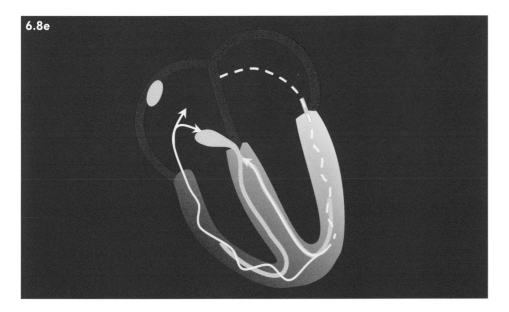

6.8e

FURTHER READING

1. Supraventricular tachycardia. In: Prystowsky EN, Klein GJ. Cardiac Arrhythmias: An Integrated Approach for the Clinician. New York: McGraw-Hill, 1994:99–130.

2. Supraventricular tachycardia. In: Josephson ME. Clinical Cardiac Electrophysiology, Second Edition. Philadelphia/London: Lea and Febiger, 1993:181–274.

3. Miles WM, Yee R, Klein GJ et al. The preexcitation index: an aid in determining the mechanism of supraventricular tachycardia and localizing accessory pathways. Circulation 1986;74(3):493–500.

4. Kerr CR, Gallagher JJ, German LD. Changes in ventriculoatrial intervals with bundle branch block aberration during reciprocating tachycardia in patients with accessory atrioventricular pathways. Circulation 1982;66(1):196–201.

5. Klein GJ, Bashore TM, Sellers TD et al. Ventricular fibrillation in the Wolff-Parkinson-White syndrome. N Engl J Med 1979;301(20):1080–5.

6. Critelli G, Gallagher JJ, Monda V et al. Anatomic and electrophysiologic substrate of the permanent form of junctional reciprocating tachycardia. J Am Coll Cardiol 1984;4(3):601–10.

7. Knight BP, Zivin A, Souza J et al. A technique for the rapid diagnosis of atrial tachycardia in the electrophysiology laboratory. J Am Coll Cardiol 1999;33(3):775–81.

7.1 PROGRAMMED VENTRICULAR STIMULATION

7.2 SIGNIFICANCE OF INDUCED VENTRICULAR ARRHYTHMIAS

7.3 SUSTAINED MONOMORPHIC VT

7.4 SPECIFIC TYPES OF VT

A wide variety of ventricular arrhythmias, associated with a range of mechanisms and clinical manifestations, are encountered in the electrophysiology (EP) laboratory. Of these, monomorphic ventricular tachycardia (VT) is of principal interest as it is the only ventricular arrhythmia that can be studied by conventional methods. EP testing is of much less value in patients with non-sustained VT, polymorphic VT (such as torsade de pointes in the long QT syndromes) or primary ventricular fibrillation.

This section will discuss the use of programmed ventricular stimulation for the induction, characterization and termination of VT. VT encountered in clinical practice is usually related to reentry around a scar, most often caused by myocardial infarction. However, three other types will also be discussed; although unusual, their recognition is important because they are generally more easily amenable than scar-related VT to catheter ablation. The techniques of mapping and ablation for these, as well as scar-related VT, will be discussed in Section 8.

The indications for EP testing in VT patients are evolving rapidly, and a dogmatic statement of these would be inappropriate here. In general, programmed ventricular stimulation is used: (i) to evaluate the inducibility of VT in patients thought to be at risk (e.g. previous VT, unexplained syncope or non-sustained ventricular arrhythmias with structural heart disease); (ii) to characterize the VT and assist in the choice of therapy; (iii) for the purposes of catheter mapping and ablation; and (iv) to evaluate the efficacy of treatment.

Extrastimulus testing is used for the induction of VT, as the rhythm generally has a reentrant mechanism. Most EP centers use a stimulation protocol in which the aggressiveness of testing is progressively increased. In the comprehensive 12-stage induction protocol described by Wellens et al., up to three ventricular extrastimuli are introduced, first in sinus rhythm, then following pacing drive trains at three different cycle lengths. With successive stages, the drive trains are made more rapid and more extrastimuli are introduced.

Most centers use an abbreviated form of this protocol, such as the following (illustrated in Figure 7.1). A quadripolar catheter paces and senses at the right ventricular apex, and a second multipolar catheter is positioned at the His position to record atrial and His bundle activity (a right atrial catheter may also be used if the need for atrial pacing is thought likely — see

Section 7.3). Following an eight-beat pacing drive train (S1) at a cycle length of 600 ms, a premature extrastimulus (S2) is introduced. This is repeated with successively shorter coupling intervals (S1S2) of the extrastimulus until VT is induced or ventricular refractoriness is reached. If VT is not induced, a second extrastimulus (S3) is introduced while S1S2 is held just

above the ventricular refractory period. S2S3 is again progressively reduced until VT is induced or refractoriness is reached. Subsequently, single (S2) and double (S2S3) extrastimuli are delivered in a similar fashion with a faster drive train (S1S1 = 400 ms). Finally, triple extrastimuli (S2S3S4) are introduced in a similar fashion after drive trains at 600 ms and 400 ms.

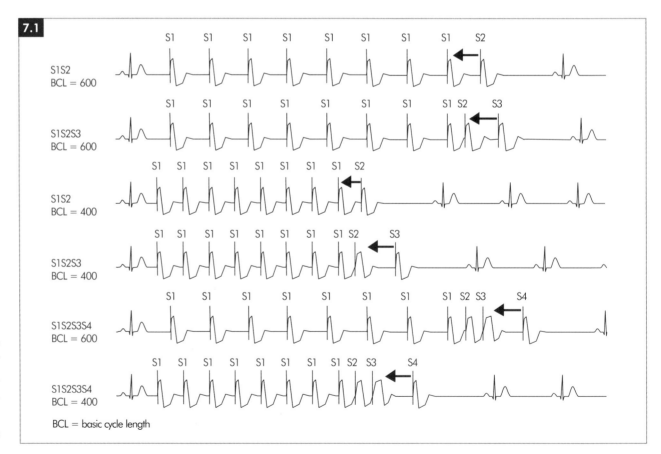

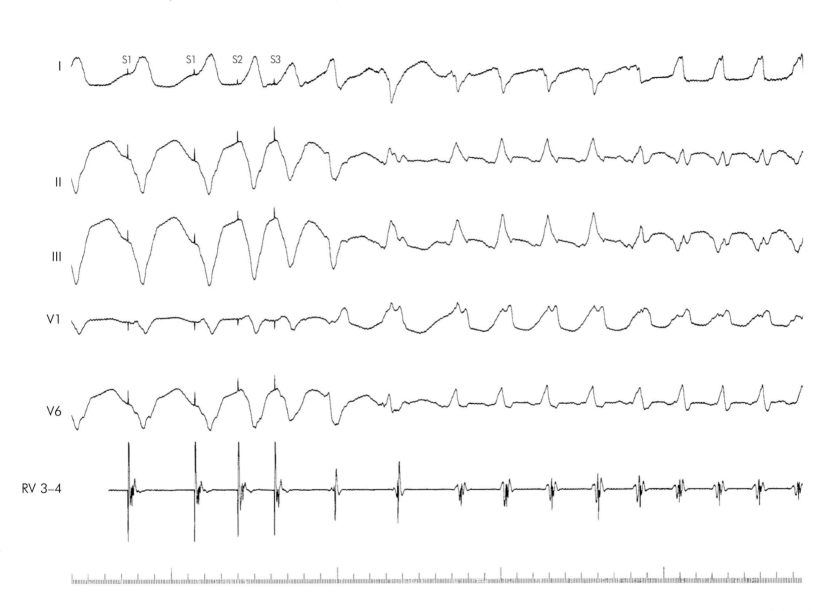

Tracing 7.1 Induction of ventricular tachycardia in a 76-year-old man with previous myocardial infarction. Right ventricular pacing at cycle length (CL) 400 ms is followed by two extrastimuli at 270 ms (S2) and 220 ms (S3) (400-270-220). By the right half of the tracing, a sustained monomorphic VT (cycle length 240 ms; similar to the clinical tachycardia) is established.

SIGNIFICANCE OF INDUCED VENTRICULAR ARRHYTHMIAS

7.2A REPETITIVE VENTRICULAR RESPONSE

Extrastimulus delivery often results in a repetitive ventricular response. This is a single or short series of ventricular beats following the extrastimulus, often with a similar morphology to the paced QRS. This phenomenon is usually attributed to reentry within the bundle branches or local myocardium, and is of no clinical significance.

7.2B SPECIFICITY OF PROGRAMMED VENTRICULAR STIMULATION

The ease of VT induction is related to the substrate (easier in infarct-related VT than cardiomyopathy) and to the aggressiveness of the stimulation protocol. The 'yield' of testing improves as additional extrastimuli are added. This gain is achieved at the expense of specificity. Sustained monomorphic VT is considered a specific finding however it is induced. The induction of non-sustained polymorphic VT or ventricular fibrillation (VF) by triple or quadruple extrastimuli may be a nonspecific finding, not necessarily related to underlying heart disease or arrhythmic risk. The induction of polymorphic VT or VF by single or double extrastimuli is in a 'grey zone' and considered specific by some. Similarly, the use of a second stimulation site (e.g. the right ventricular outflow tract or the left ventricle) and the infusion of isoproterenol during testing improve sensitivity but at the expense of specificity.

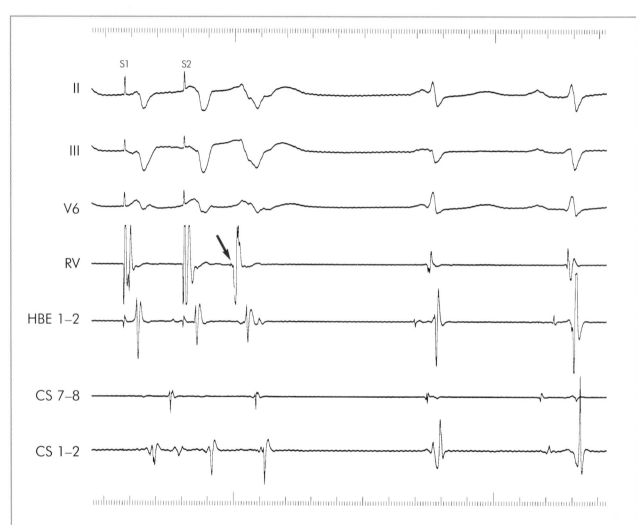

Tracing 7.2a A single repetitive ventricular response follows a closely-coupled extrastimulus (S2). The morphology of the repetitive ventricular response is almost identical to that of the paced beats. As the repetitive response originates near the catheter tip, the right ventricular electrogram comes at the beginning of the QRS deflection (arrow).

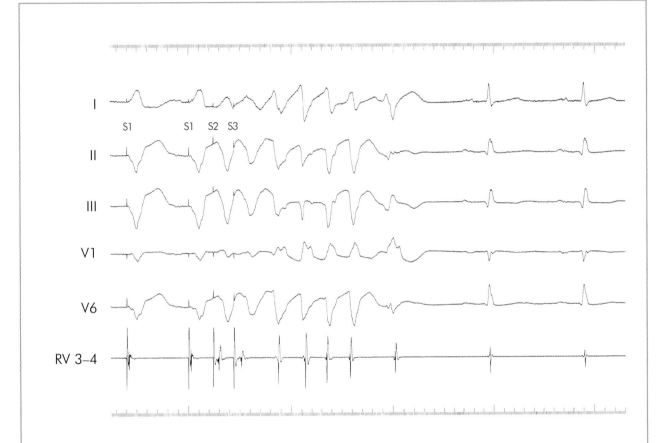

I

S1   S1 S2 S3

II

III

V1

V6

RV 3–4

Tracing 7.2b Induction of non-sustained polymorphic VT. Right ventricular pacing (cycle length 600 ms) is followed by two extrastimuli at 230 ms (S2) and 200 ms (S3) (600-230-200). Induction of non-sustained polymorphic VT with multiple closely-coupled extrastimuli.

For the purpose of risk assessment, it is our practice to limit testing to the use of three extrastimuli at two drive cycle lengths and two stimulation sites. However, if the purpose of EP testing is to induce a known arrhythmia so that it can be studied or ablated, we use more aggressive methods as necessary.

Some forms of idiopathic VT (see Section 7.4) differ from VT associated with structural heart disease. Notably, with idiopathic right ventricular outflow tract (RVOT) (see Section 7.4B), macro-reentry is not the mechanism and extrastimulus testing is therefore of limited use for VT induction. Adjuncts used to facilitate automaticity include isoproterenol, epinephrine, atropine and exercise. Triggered activity may be induced with multiple extrastimuli, burst pacing or long-short stimulus sequences, accompanied by the above drugs and possibly aminophylline or calcium.

Once a sustained monomorphic wide-complex tachycardia has been induced, a full 12-lead surface ECG should be recorded immediately. Even if the arrhythmia causes significant hemodynamic deterioration, there is usually time to record an ECG while preparing for cardioversion. The surface ECG can be used for comparison with recordings of spontaneous VT (to determine whether the induced tachycardia is the same), and may be useful for pace-mapping (see Section 8.4). The intracardiac electrograms should also be recorded.

If the arrhythmia does not require immediate cardioversion, programmed stimulation can be used to further characterize the VT and attempt pace termination. It should be possible to answer the following questions.

7.3A   IS IT VT?

The differential diagnosis of a wide complex (>120 ms) tachycardia is: (i) supraventricular origin, with aberrant conduction (usually a typical bundle branch block); (ii) supraventricular origin, with ventricular pre-excitation (see Section 6.8); and (iii) VT. A number of pieces of evidence support the diagnosis of VT: (i) inducibility from the ventricle but not the atrium; (ii) QRS morphology that is highly atypical for bundle branch block or pre-excitation; and (iii) lack of response to adenosine. However, these do not constitute proof; the key to a positive diagnosis of VT is the demonstration that the atria are not part of the tachycardia mechanism. In at least two-thirds of cases, retrograde conduction over the AV node is absent during VT, and ventriculoatrial (VA) dissociation is observed. If 1:1 VA conduction is present, atrial pacing may be of help: if the atria can be dissociated while the tachycardia continues unaffected, a diagnosis of VT is made, with rare exceptions.

7.3B   WHAT ARE THE CLINICAL AND ECG CHARACTERISTICS?

Whenever sustained monomorphic VT is induced, it should be characterized in terms of its cycle length, hemodynamic effects, morphology and axis. A tachycardia that is slow and well tolerated hemodynamically is more likely to be amenable to pace-termination and catheter ablation than one that causes collapse. As a rule, the QRS morphology in VT is different from that in typical bundle branch block. However, VT is described as having 'right bundle branch block' (RBBB) morphology if the terminal portion of the QRS complex in V1 is positive, and as having 'left bundle branch block' (LBBB) morphology if this is negative.

Together with the frontal plane axis, the QRS morphology can give a first approximation to the location of the tachycardia origin. As seen in Figure 7.3b, RBBB morphology suggests activation arising from the left ventricle or septum, while LBBB morphology is usually seen in VT arising from the right ventricle. An inferior axis suggests activation from the base of the heart (especially the outflow tracts), and a superior axis or one beyond 90° suggests activation from near the apex.

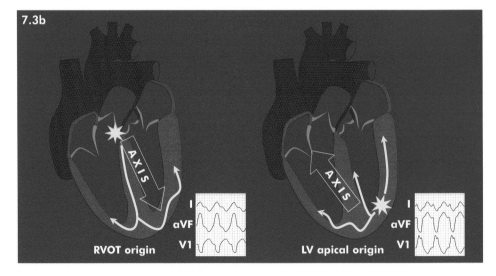

7.3b

RVOT origin

LV apical origin

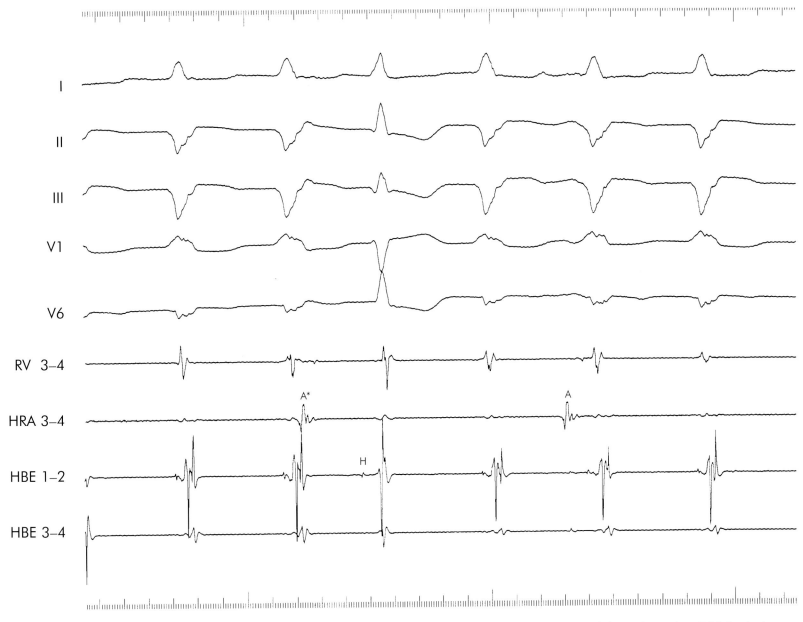

Tracing 7.3a Sustained monomorphic VT in a 72-year-old man with two previous myocardial infarctions and congestive heart failure. The surface ECG leads show a wide-complex tachycardia with RBBB morphology and left axis QRS morphology (cycle length 440 ms). The right atrial catheter (HRA) records sinus rhythm confirming AV dissociation. The third QRS complex is narrow and premature; it is a capture beat resulting from conduction of the sinus beat seen in the HRA (A*) via the His bundle (H).

7.3C WHAT IS THE RELATIONSHIP BETWEEN VENTRICULAR AND HIS ACTIVATION?

The relationship between activation of the His bundle and that of the ventricles is critical to the diagnosis of bundle branch reentry (see Section 7.4D). If this mechanism is suspected, it is important to obtain a clear His recording, and another catheter may be used to record from the right bundle branch. Ventricular or atrial extrastimuli may be introduced to 'disturb' the tachycardia and determine whether changes in His activation precede or follow changes in ventricular activation.

7.3D HOW CAN THE ARRHYTHMIA BE TERMINATED?

If VT causes hemodynamic collapse, synchronized cardioversion should be performed. Many operators prefer to wait a few seconds until the patient has become fully unconscious before delivering a shock, and most give an intravenous sedative with amnestic properties, such as midazolam.

If VT is well tolerated, the operator should attempt pace-termination. Easy termination of VT by timed ventricular extrastimuli suggests a macro-reentrant mechanism with a large excitable gap. Burst pacing initially a little faster than the tachycardia, then repeated at progressively shorter cycle lengths until VT is interrupted, is simpler and usually effective. Ramp pacing (a feature of implantable defibrillators in which a sequence of stimuli are separated by progressively shorter intervals) may also be used. The more aggressive the pacing intervention, the more likely it is to accelerate rather than terminate the VT. The results of pacing intervention may be useful for the selection and programming of implantable cardioverter-defibrillator therapy.

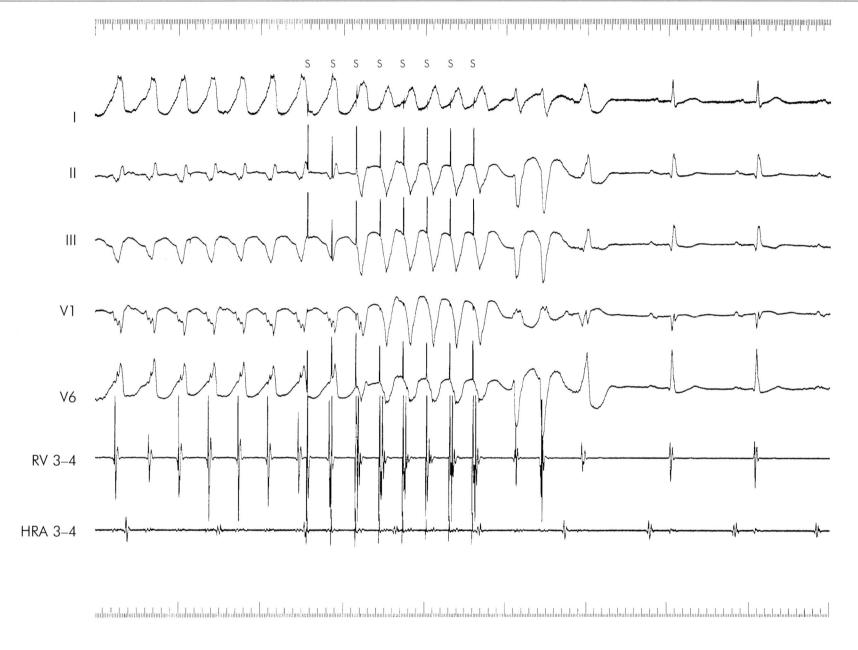

Tracing 7.3d Pace-termination in a patient with sustained monomorphic VT (cycle length 360 ms). An eight-beat pacing burst (cycle length 280 ms) is delivered, followed by two repetitive ventricular responses and resumption of sinus rhythm.

Common forms of VT seen in the EP lab are listed in Table 1. Those that are associated with structural heart disease are usually caused by macro-reentry based on slow conduction through diseased ventricular myocardium. Tachycardia can generally be induced and often terminated by programmed ventricular stimulation; if necessary, the reentrant mechanism can be proven using entrainment techniques (see Sections 3 and 8). In contrast, idiopathic VT may be associated with enhanced automaticity (e.g. right ventricular outflow tract VT) or triggered activity. Routine extrastimulus testing may be ineffective at initiating these types of VT in the EP laboratory; long-short pacing sequences and burst pacing may be useful, but pharmacological provocation and a degree of luck are often necessary.

TABLE 1   FORMS OF VT

VT associated with structural heart disease

> Infarct-related
> Dilated cardiomyopathy
> Hypertrophic cardiomyopathy
> Arrhythmogenic right ventricular cardiomyopathy
> Bundle branch reentry

Idiopathic VT

> Right ventricular outflow tract (RVOT)
> Idiopathic left ventricle VT
> Miscellaneous (left ventricular outflow tract (LVOT), RV free wall)

7.4A   SCAR-RELATED VT

The overwhelming majority of VT seen in the developed world is related to prior myocardial infarction. The classical ingredients for reentry (see Section 3.4) are present; a scar provides the central obstacle around which the circuit revolves, and the peri-infarct zone, containing islands of viable myocytes within fibrous scar tissue, provides the slow-conducting substrate. Critically-timed premature ventricular complexes (either spontaneous or provided by the electrophysiologist) initiate and terminate tachycardia. VT associated with other forms of structural heart disease (e.g. hypertrophic and dilated cardiomyopathy, arrhythmogenic right ventricular cardiomyopathy) are thought to have similar mechanisms, with the substrate provided by less discrete scarring or myocardial disarray. Infarct-related VT (e.g. Tracing 7.3a) can have any morphology or axis, though typically the QRS complex is very wide (>140 ms). A left ventricular origin (i.e. RBBB) is somewhat more common than a right ventricular origin, and a 'normal' axis, implying origin from the outflow tracts, is less common than an abnormal axis.

7.4a

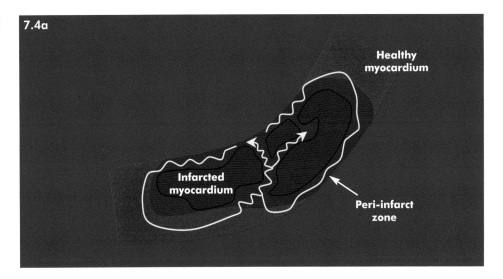

Healthy myocardium

Infarcted myocardium

Peri-infarct zone

7.4B RIGHT VENTRICULAR OUTFLOW TRACT VT

RVOT tachycardia is the commonest form of idiopathic VT. The typical pattern is of frequent unifocal premature ventricular complexes arising from the RVOT, having an LBBB morphology and an inferior axis (Figure 7.3b, left). With exercise or stress, these can be transformed to salvos or sustained tachycardia (Tracing 7.4b). Termination by adenosine and a degree of suppressibility by β-blockade are the rule. If the heart is structurally normal, the arrhythmia is thought to be benign, but catheter ablation should be considered for symptomatic patients. The major differential diagnosis is reentrant tachycardia due to arrhythmogenic RV cardiomyopathy (best detected by magnetic resonance imaging). Catheter ablation for RVOT VT has a high success rate, but the major limitation is the frequent inability to induce tachycardia in the EP laboratory. Because the presumed mechanism is triggered activity rather than reentry, isoproterenol or epinephrine may facilitate induction, and neuroleptic sedation is preferred over general anesthesia. Activation mapping (see Section 8.4B) is generally more accurate than pace-mapping (see Section 8.4A), but the latter can be useful when tachycardia is not sustained. A much less common left ventricular outflow tract form of VT has also been described.

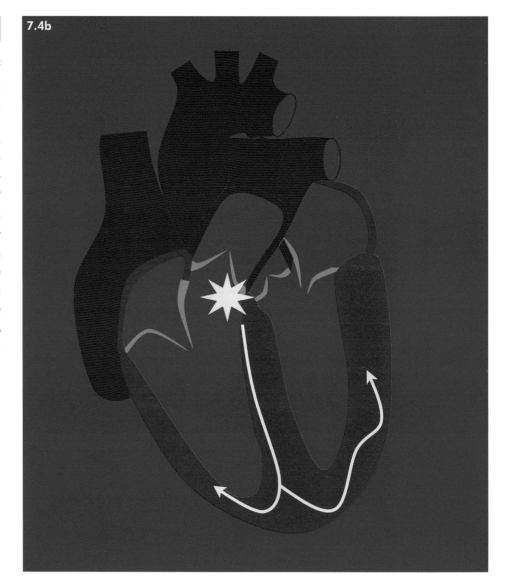

7.4b

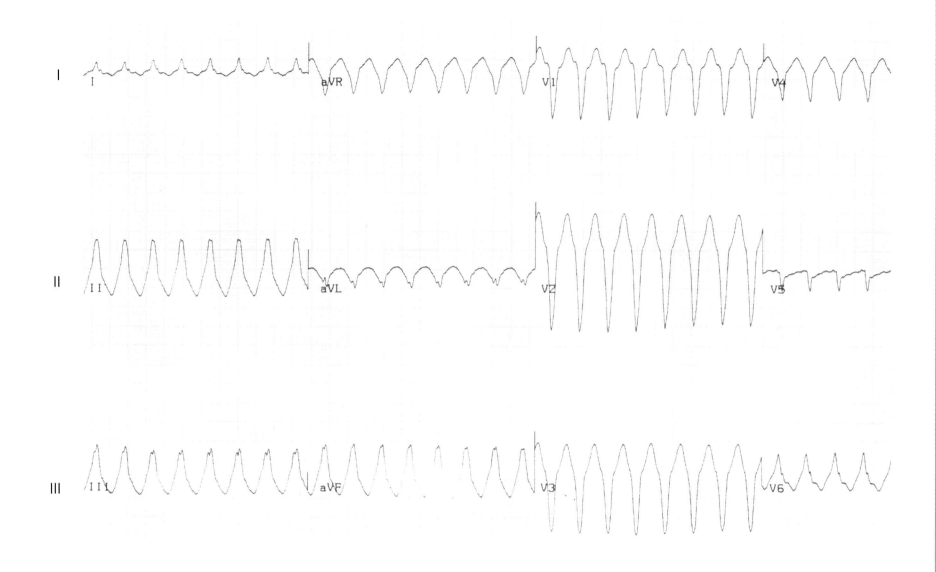

Tracing 7.4b RVOT VT. The morphology resembles LBBB and the axis is inferior.

7.4C   IDIOPATHIC LEFT VENTRICULAR TACHYCARDIA

Idiopathic left ventricular tachycardia (previously known as 'fascicular VT') is characterized by sensitivity to verapamil. Induction may be facilitated by isoproterenol or atropine, or a bolus of intravenous calcium chloride. This tachycardia has a right bundle branch block and left axis QRS morphology (Tracing 7.4c). Echocardiography demonstrates normal left ventricular function, and an LV moderator band is frequently seen. The mechanism has been the subject of speculation, and was thought to be triggered activity. However, the tachycardia now appears to be caused by reentry with a slowly conducting 'diastolic' segment along the left ventricular aspect of the interventricular septum. The ventricle is activated from the exit point of this diastolic segment, in the posteroapical part of the septum. Catheter ablation is traditionally generally guided by activation- and/or pace-mapping to identify the exit point from which ventricular activation spreads. At this location, the early ventricular electrogram is usually preceded by a sharp fascicular potential. An alternative, and possibly more successful, ablation strategy is to identify diastolic potentials arising nearer the entrance to the diastolic segment of the circuit high in the septum.

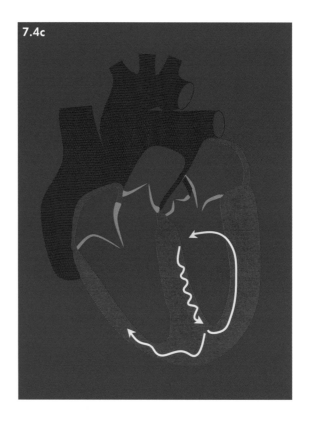

7.4c

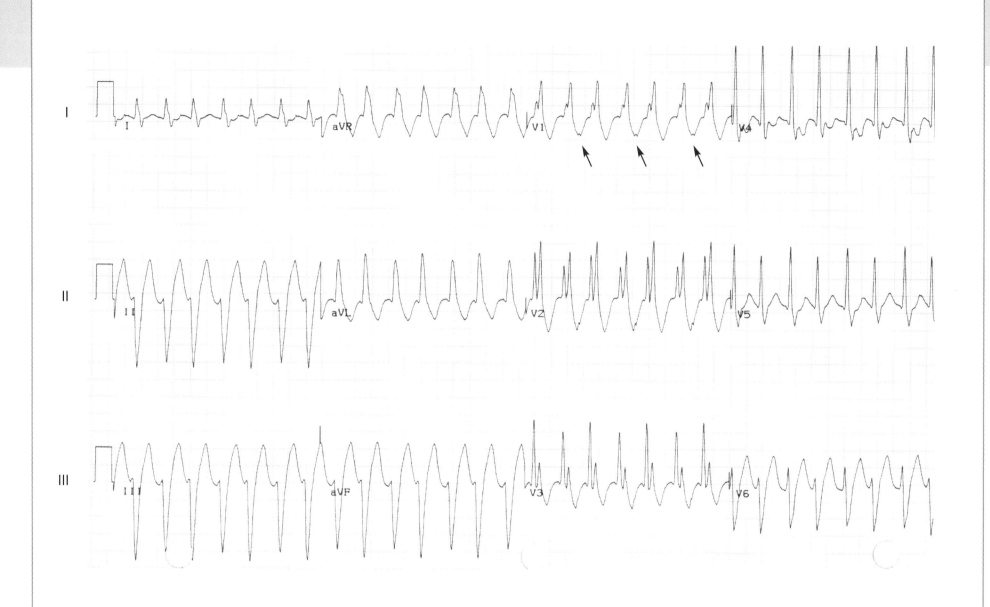

Tracing 7.4c Fascicular tachycardia. The morphology resembles RBBB and the axis is superior. Note the 2:1 V:A ratio (P-waves, arrowed, distort every other T-wave in V1 and V2).

7.4D BUNDLE BRANCH REENTRY

Bundle branch reentrant tachycardia is caused by a macro-reentrant circuit around the two sides of the interventricular septum. It is most commonly seen in patients with LV dilatation and partial or complete LBBB with a long PR interval in sinus rhythm (Figure 7.4d-i). Slow conduction around a long circuit path is necessary for reentry to be possible.

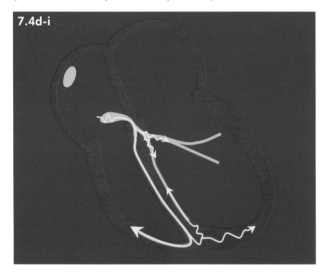

7.4d-i

As shown in Figure 7.4d-ii, following unidirectional block in the left bundle, activation proceeds down the right bundle, across the septum, and up the left bundle to complete the circuit at the bifurcation of the His bundle. The ECG in tachycardia typically has an LBBB morphology with a leftward axis because

activation arises from the distal right bundle. A prolonged HV interval is usually noted in sinus rhythm, which may shorten, remain unchanged or prolong during tachycardia, depending on the relative positioning of the His recording catheter to the bifurcation of the bundle branch system and the conduction time of the right bundle. His recording demonstrates that changes in the His-to-His interval precede and predict the subsequent V-to-V interval.

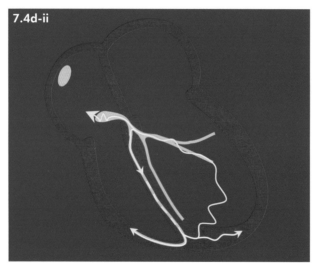

7.4d-ii

TABLE 2 DIAGNOSTIC CRITERIA FOR BUNDLE BRANCH REENTRY

Typical LBBB or RBBB morphology during tachycardia

Each ventricular activation is preceded by His bundle activation, with a stable HV interval

Variations in VV interval are preceded and predicted by variations in HH interval

Tachycardia induction depends on critical delay in the His-Purkinje system

Tachycardia is terminated by block in the His-Purkinje system

Tachycardia is abolished by ablation of the right bundle branch

Although the commonest pattern of bundle branch reentry is that described above, the reverse tachycardia (with RBBB morphology) can be seen, as can (occasionally) reentry between the divisions of the left bundle. Bundle branch reentry is an uncommon but important form of VT because ablation of the right bundle can be curative. This may create the need for permanent pacing due to AV block.

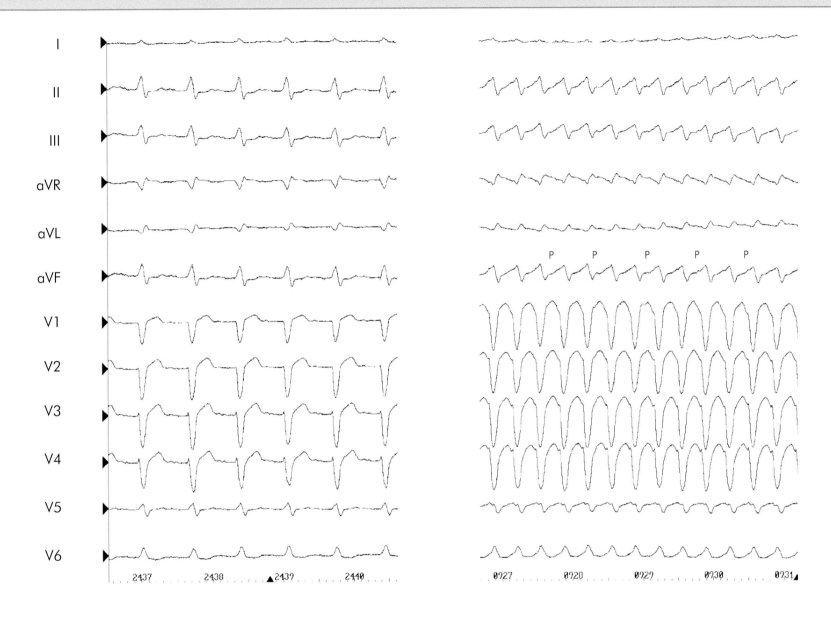

Tracing 7.4d-i 12-lead ECGs from a patient with dilated cardiomyopathy. In sinus rhythm (left), there is LBBB with marked PR prolongation, suggestive of extensive conduction tissue disease. During tachycardia (right), the QRS morphology is virtually identical, indicating that ventricular activation is the same as in sinus rhythm. This would normally suggest supraventricular tachycardia with aberrant conduction, but in this case the diagnosis of VT is confirmed by the presence of dissociated P-waves. This combination of history and ECG findings is highly suggestive of bundle branch reentry. (Courtesy of Dr MA Barlow.)

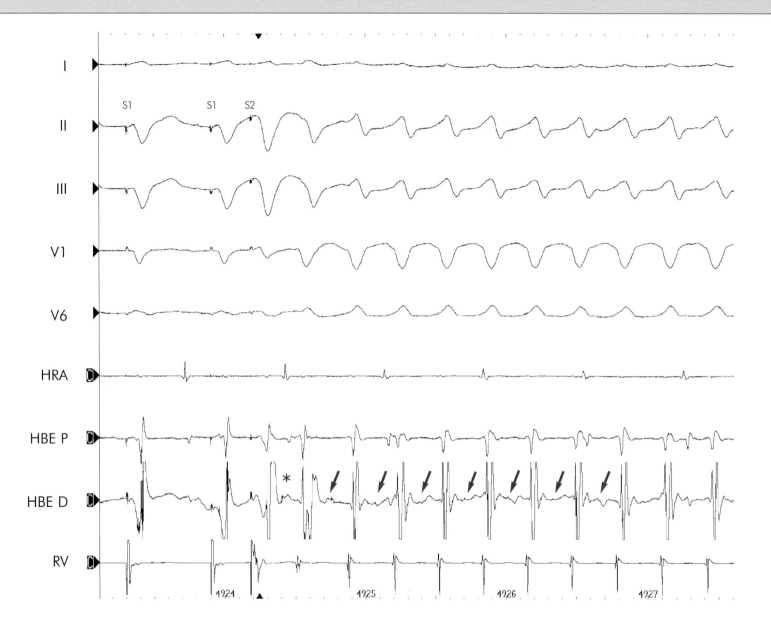

Tracing 7.4d-ii Induction of bundle branch reentrant VT. Following a ventricular extrastimulus (S2), delay in the VH interval reveals a His potential (*) after the ventricular electrogram. In subsequent beats, each His potential (arrow) has a fixed relationship to the following ventricular electrogram. (Courtesy of Dr MA Barlow.)

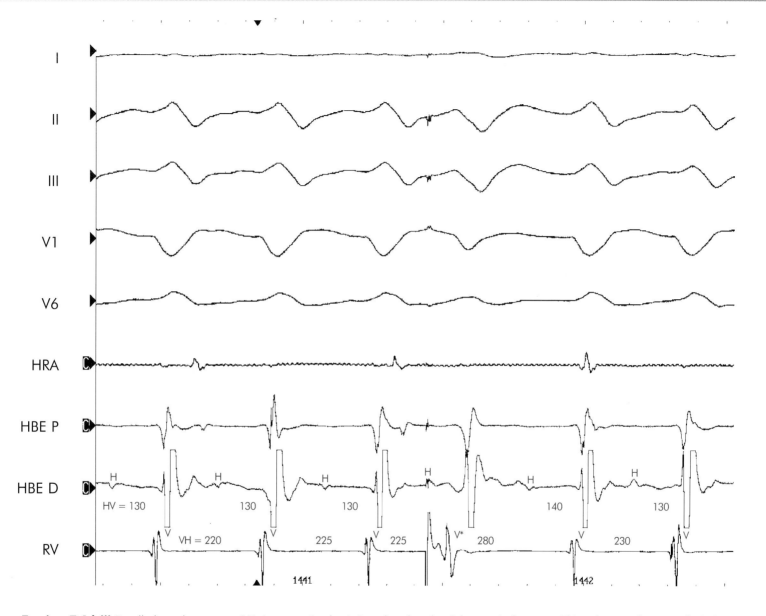

Tracing 7.4d-iii Bundle branch reentrant VT. An extrastimulus is introduced at the right ventricular apex. This advances the ventricle (V*) and slightly advances the tachycardia. Through this perturbation, the HV interval (conduction over the RBB) remains constant, while the variability is in the VH interval (ventricular myocardium and LBB) – compare the V*H interval following the extrastimulus to the other VH intervals. (Courtesy of Dr MA Barlow.)

FURTHER READING

1. Ventricular tachycardias. In: Zipes DP, Jalife J. Cardiac Electrophysiology: From Cell to Bedside. Philadelphia: WB Saunders, 1999: 530–54 and 640–55.

2. Ventricular tachycardia. In: Prystowsky EN, Klein GJ. Cardiac Arrhythmias: An Integrated Approach for the Clinician. New York: McGraw-Hill, 1994:155–77.

3. Recurrent ventricular tachycardia. In: Josephson ME. Clinical Cardiac Electrophysiology, Second Edition. Philadelphia/London: Lea and Febiger, 1993:417–615.

4. Wellens HJ, Bar FW, Lie KI. The value of the electrocardiogram in the differential diagnosis of a tachycardia with a widened QRS complex. Am J Med 1978;64(1):27–33.

5. Wellens HJ, Brugada P, Stevenson WG. Programmed electrical stimulation of the heart in patients with life-threatening ventricular arrhythmias: what is the significance of induced arrhythmias and what is the correct protocol. Circulation 1985;72:1–7.

6. Frazier DW, Stanton MS. Resetting and transient entrainment of ventricular tachycardia. Pacing Clin Electrophysiol 1995;18(10):1919–46.

7. Stevenson WG, Friedman PL, Kocovic D et al. Radiofrequency catheter ablation of ventricular tachycardia after myocardial infarction. Circulation 1998;98(4):308–14.

8. Delacretaz E, Stevenson WG, Ellison KE et al. Mapping and radiofrequency catheter ablation of the three types of sustained monomorphic ventricular tachycardia in nonischemic heart disease. J Cardiovasc Electrophysiol 2000;11(1):11–7.

9. Blanck Z, Sra J, Dhala A et al. Bundle branch reentry: mechanisms, diagnosis, and treatment. In: Zipes DP, Jalife J. Cardiac Electrophysiology: From Cell to Bedside. Philadelphia: WB Saunders, 1999: 656–61.

10. Tchou P, Mehdirad AA. Bundle branch reentry ventricular tachycardia. Pacing Clin Electrophysiol 1995;18(7):1427–37.

MAPPING AND CATHETER ABLATION   8

The techniques of catheter ablation are difficult to learn from a book: there is no substitute for practical experience in a teaching environment. This section will therefore concentrate on the principles of ablation, with particular reference to mapping and the characteristics of ablation electrograms. The practicalities of catheter selection and manipulation will not be discussed in detail.

First, we will briefly discuss the physics of direct current shock and radiofrequency energy delivery, and the reasons that the latter is the current choice for catheter ablation. Second, we will describe the principles behind different types of ablation procedure, according to the type of arrhythmia substrate:

(i)   ablation of fixed structures using anatomical landmarks and electrogram morphology (atrioventricular (AV) nodal ablation and modification)
(ii) mapping and ablation of tachycardias with a 'focal' origin (ectopic atrial and certain ventricular tachycardias)
(iii) mapping and ablation of accessory AV pathways
(iv) ablation of an anatomically defined macro-reentrant circuit (typical atrial flutter)
(v)   mapping and ablation of unknown macro-reentrant circuits (scar-related ventricular tachycardia and atypical flutter)

Finally, we will briefly discuss some experimental alternative energy sources and catheter designs for ablation, and emerging computerized mapping technologies.

8.1A   DIRECT CURRENT SHOCK

The first transvenous catheter ablations, performed in the early 1980s, used direct current (DC) shocks to destroy the AV node and achieve complete heart block. With this technique, a capacitor discharge of 200–300 J is delivered between a catheter positioned by the AV node in the right atrium and an indifferent skin patch (Figure 8.1a-i).

Typically, the pulse has a leading edge of 1–3 kV and a duration of approximately 5 ms. During the first 2 ms, a current of up to 40 A causes heating of blood and myocardium. After approximately 2 ms, there is a sharp rise in impedance, as blood heating causes a flash of plasma arc and an explosive steam bubble to form. At this point, current drops sharply and ceases for approximately 0.5 ms. A shockwave accompanies collapse of the steam bubble approximately 5 ms after the onset of the shock (Figure 8.1a-ii).

Most myocardial necrosis is caused by the current during the first 2 ms, while barotrauma from the explosion that follows can occasionally lead to rupture of myocardial structures, hypotension and arrhythmias. For this reason, 'low energy' DC shocks (up to 40 J delivered) have been used – these use a truncated pulse waveform to retain the high initial voltage and current while avoiding arcing and barotrauma.

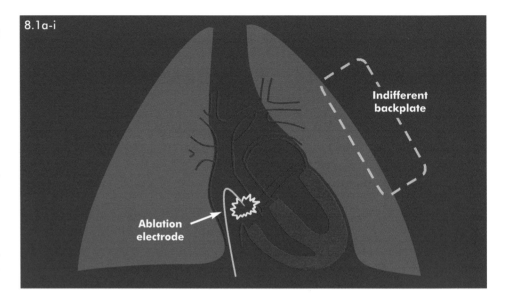

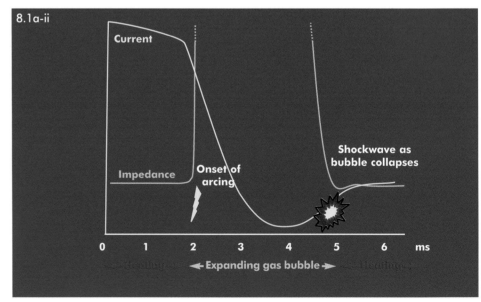

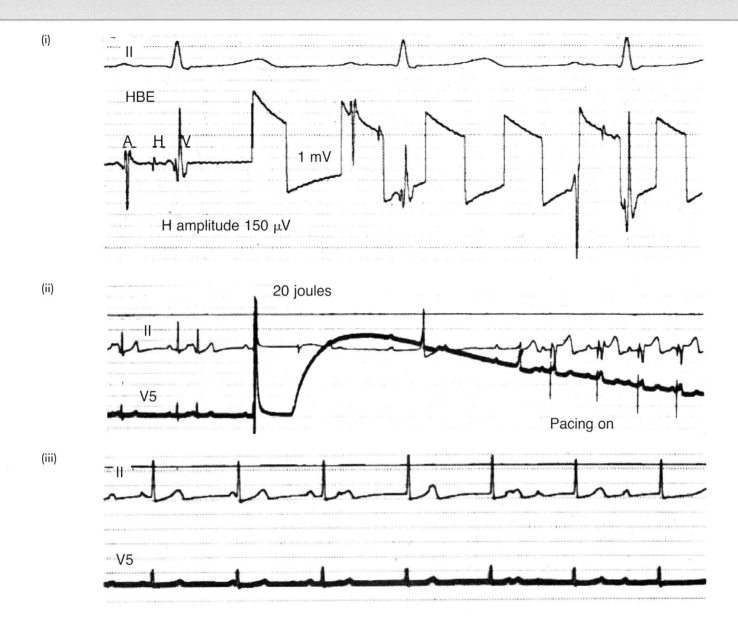

(i)

II

HBE

A H V

1 mV

H amplitude 150 µV

(ii)

20 joules

II

V5

Pacing on

(iii)

II

V5

Tracing 8.1a AV nodal ablation using a low energy DC shock, from before the era of radiofrequency ablation. (i) Signals recorded at the ablation location show balanced atrial and ventricular electrograms, with a sharp His deflection (the calibration signal was used to measure the His amplitude). (ii) A 20 J truncated shock is delivered synchronous to the QRS complex, and results in complete AV block. Pacing is instituted after a few seconds. (iii) The final outcome is complete heart block with a junctional escape rhythm. (Courtesy of Dr Edward Rowland, St George's Hospital Medical School, London.)

8.1B   RADIOFREQUENCY ENERGY

Radiofrequency (RF) ablation uses alternating current delivered between the catheter tip and an indifferent electrode (again, usually a skin patch) to achieve tissue necrosis. The choice of frequency and pulse form is important for both safety and efficacy. RF current (generally 300–750 kHz) does not cause direct myocardial depolarization and is therefore free of the risk of fibrillation that is present with lower frequencies (e.g. 50 Hz). The RF current used in electrosurgery is delivered in high voltage (~1 kV), short pulses (~4 ms), which promote arcing and coagulation (Figure 8.1b-i). Conversely, that used for catheter ablation is continuous, and uses a low voltage (typically 40 V) – this causes controlled thermal injury to the tissue by two mechanisms.

Resistive heating is caused directly by the electrical current producing oscillations of ions in solution. This only directly affects tissue close (~1 mm) to the electrode interface, as the power delivered to the myocardium is inversely proportional to the fourth power of the distance from the electrode. However, heat is conducted from this small area to adjacent tissue, and this *conductive heating* is responsible for the majority of the thermal injury (Figure 8.1b-ii).

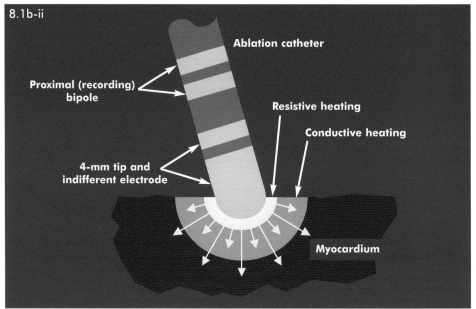

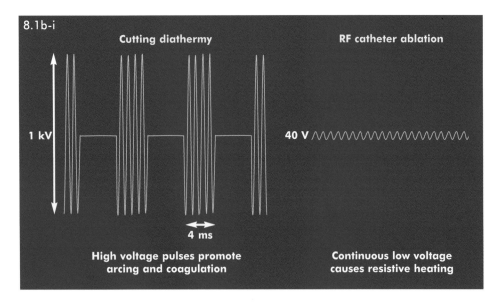

RF ablation offers a number of advantages over DC shock: the lesion created is discrete, and its location is precisely defined with minimal risk of damage to adjacent structures. Perhaps most importantly, the lesion is created over a period of time. Irreversible injury occurs when myocardial tissue reaches a temperature around 48–50°C. It generally takes between 5 and 20 s for a steady-state to be achieved between current delivery and heat dissipation by tissue and blood.

During this time, the electrophysiological effects can be continuously monitored. If a desired result (e.g. block in an accessory pathway) is seen within a few seconds, the location is deemed appropriate and energy delivery is continued for at least 30 s. Conversely, if an adverse result (e.g. unwanted effects on AV nodal conduction) is seen, or if the catheter is moved inadvertently, energy delivery can quickly be discontinued with the hope of avoiding permanent damage.

In most cases, when successful ablation has been achieved, the result is permanent. However, it is not uncommon to see the return of conduction in a pathway, or recurrence of a focal arrhythmia, a few minutes after ablation. This is presumably due to injury rather than necrosis to the critical tissue. For this reason, electrophysiologists sometimes deliver an extra burn to expand the lesion at a successful ablation site. It is our practice to monitor the patient for 30 mins, following an apparently successful ablation, before conducting final electrophysiological testing: recurrence after that time is highly unusual.

8.1C TEMPERATURE CONTROL DURING RADIOFREQUENCY ABLATION

The size of the RF lesion needed in ablation depends on the arrhythmia substrate. A power of 30 W delivered to a 4-mm tip catheter typically creates a lesion approximately 4–5 mm in diameter and depth, which is adequate for most accessory pathway ablations and AV node modifications. The power requirements may differ in some locations. If heat dissipation by blood flowing past the tip is low (in venous structures, for example), very high surface temperatures may be reached, causing potentially dangerous gas formation and charring at the electrode interface. The resulting impedance rise is detected by the RF energy generator, and energy is cut off automatically. This and the high impedance prevent an adequate lesion from being created. Conversely, some thicker structures may require greater power delivery – this is frequently the case with isthmus ablation for atrial flutter, or ablation of ventricular myocardium. Again, the limiting factor is the temperature at which impedance rises. For this reason, most ablation systems now use an electronic servo mechanism that automatically adjusts output to achieve a desired temperature. A typical setting might be 60°C, but somewhat higher temperatures may be required to achieve sufficient lesion depth. The thermistor or thermocouple in the catheter tip is close to, but not at, the electrode-tissue interface, so the measured temperature generally underestimates the actual temperature of the tissue that is being resistively heated. However, as long as the system prevents the tissue interface from reaching 100°C, gas formation and charring will be avoided.

8.2A TECHNIQUE

Catheter ablation of the AV node, to cause complete AV block, is chiefly used in patients with permanent atrial fibrillation (AF) and poorly controlled ventricular rates. The principal goal is an improvement in quality of life due to a reduction in tachycardia-related symptoms, but a hemodynamic improvement may also occur. A successful result eliminates the need for antiarrhythmic drugs, but creates life-long pacemaker dependence. The procedure is therefore best suited to older patients for whom it is a simple treatment, necessitating a very brief hospital stay, with an excellent outcome. Conversely, it is generally considered a treatment of last resort in younger patients. AV node ablation is also frequently performed for patients with drug-refractory symptoms from paroxysmal AF. However, the benefits in such patients are less firmly established, and alternative drug-based and non-pharmacological treatments are rapidly evolving. In very rare cases, AV node ablation is employed to control symptoms arising from other atrial arrhythmias that are not amenable to specific treatment.

AV node ablation is often referred to as 'His bundle' ablation. However, the therapeutic goal is to create block in the AV node itself, rather than in the His-Purkinje system. The latter usually provides a 'junctional' escape rhythm around 40 beats/min – although this does not obviate the need for ventricular pacing, it provides a useful safety backup. The procedure requires a steerable catheter for mapping and ablation, and a second catheter to pace the right ventricle once heart block is achieved.

As described in Section 4, the compact AV node lies between the center and the apex of Koch's triangle (Figure 8.2a). In most cases, it can be located by positioning the ablation catheter at the site giving the best His bundle electrogram, then withdrawing it, roughly parallel to the tricuspid annulus, by ~1 cm. A location is sought where the atrial and ventricular electrograms are of comparable amplitude,

and the His potential is just visible. If the ablation is performed in AF, it is sometimes not possible to identify the His electrogram, and anatomical landmarks are instead used. Allowance must also be made for the lower amplitude of atrial electrograms in AF compared with sinus rhythm.

The anatomy of the AV node varies considerably between patients. Even at the successful site, complete heart block may take 10–20 s or more of RF energy to occur. If energy delivery at the location described above is unsuccessful, a more aggressive approach may be necessary, aiming nearer the His bundle itself. Occasionally, it is necessary to ablate the His bundle from the left side, using a retrograde aortic approach.

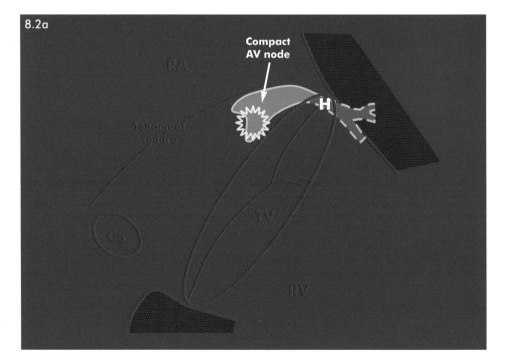

8.2a

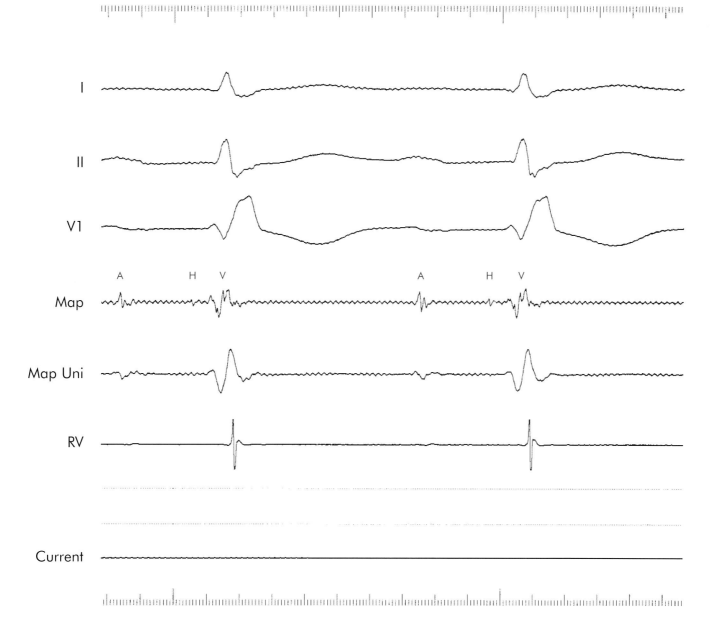

Tracing 8.2a-i Magnified ablation electrogram prior to successful current application for AV node ablation. The atrial and ventricular electrograms are of comparable amplitude, and a very small His deflection is seen.

(ii)

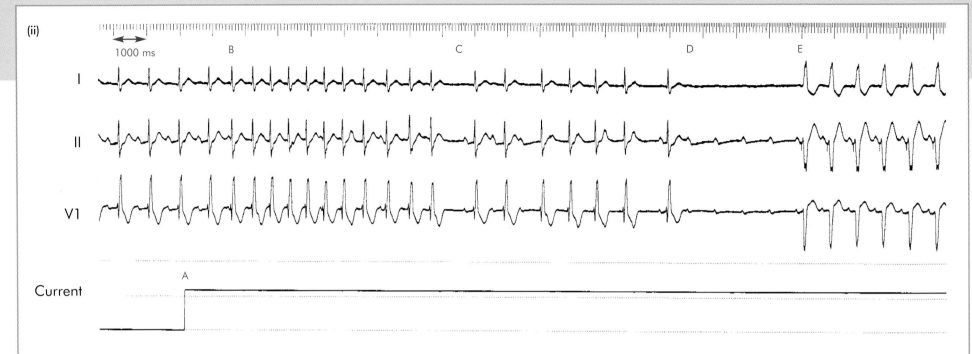

Tracing 8.2a-ii The response to AV node ablation seen on the surface ECG. Sinus rhythm with right bundle branch block (RBBB) is seen at baseline. Within seconds of the onset of current application (A), junctional tachycardia is seen (B). This gradually slows, and is followed by a period of Wenckebach AV block (C). Finally, complete AV block occurs without an escape rhythm (D), and ventricular pacing is switched on (E).

(iii)

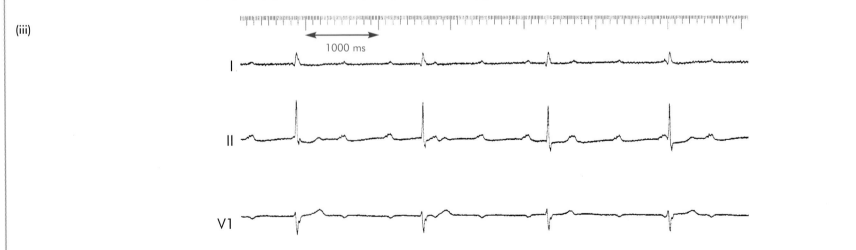

Tracing 8.2a-iii Surface ECG leads after AV node ablation showing complete AV block with junctional escape rhythm of cycle length ~1680 ms (36 beats/min).

8.2B   PACING AFTER AV NODE ABLATION

The choice of pacemaker mode after AV node ablation is dependent on patient factors: for those with permanent AF, an atrial lead is redundant and ventricular rate-responsive (VVIR) pacing is usual. Those with paroxysmal AF may benefit from a dual chamber (DDD) system that can provide AV synchrony during periods of sinus rhythm, and 'mode-switch' to a demand ventricular mode (e.g. VVIR) when atrial tachyarrhythmias are detected.

As AV nodal ablation renders patients pacing-dependent, it is essential to confirm reliable ventricular pacing before hospital discharge. In some centers, AV nodal ablation is performed a month or two after pacemaker implantation. At this stage, lead displacement is very rare. RF energy delivery at the AV node does not seem to affect pacemaker or lead function, but a pacemaker check should be performed after the procedure anyway. This two-step strategy has two other advantages: a few patients' symptoms are sufficiently improved by pacing alone so that AV node ablation is no longer necessary; and each procedure can often be performed as a day case, without the need for an overnight stay.

A very small incidence of unexpected cardiac arrest or sudden death has been reported following AV node ablation, without evidence of pacemaker malfunction or lead displacement. This occurrence seems to have been limited to those patients in whom sustained rapid ventricular rates pre-ablation were immediately allowed to fall to normal or low rates. Though firm evidence is lacking, polymorphic ventricular tachycardia related to the adaptation of ventricular repolarization to a slower, paced rhythm – a form of acquired long QT syndrome – is a possible culprit. Therefore, many centers now program pacemakers to a lower rate ≥ 80 beats/min for the first few weeks after AV node ablation. This precaution may be unnecessary if the patient is in sinus rhythm or has a well controlled ventricular rate at the time of ablation.

In theory, a number of locations could be used as targets for catheter ablation of AV nodal reentrant tachycardia (AVNRT): the upper and lower turnaround points of the tachycardia circuit, and its two limbs (the 'fast' and 'slow' pathways). The compact AV node itself is clearly part of the circuit, and was the original target for surgical and catheter-based ablation. This, however, necessarily produced AV block. Subsequently, it was found that surgical destruction of perinodal tissue could eliminate AVNRT yet leave AV conduction intact — the concept of 'fast' and 'slow' inputs to the node arose from this finding (see Section 4.4). The upper turnaround portion of the circuit is presumably in the atrial tissue, though its path remains unclear. Catheter ablation is therefore directed at the fast or slow pathway, and nowadays almost always the latter.

8.3A 'FAST PATHWAY' ABLATION

As described in Section 4.4, the 'fast pathway' is generally anteroseptal (properly, superior) to the His electrogram (Figure 8.3a). A successful fast pathway ablation causes an increase in the AH and therefore the PR interval, as conduction is now solely over the slow pathway, and AVNRT is impossible. Retrograde conduction through the node is usually fast-pathway dependent and therefore abolished. This was the method originally used for AV nodal modification, but AV block was a rather frequent complication, and the slow pathway approach is now preferred.

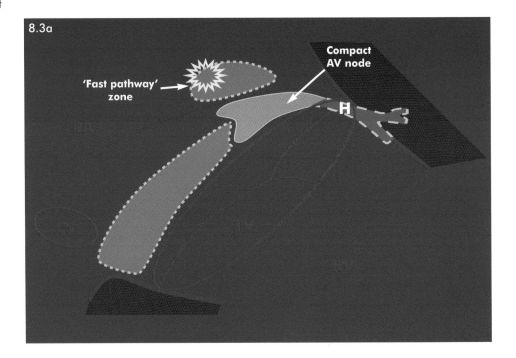

8.3a

'Fast pathway' zone

Compact AV node

H

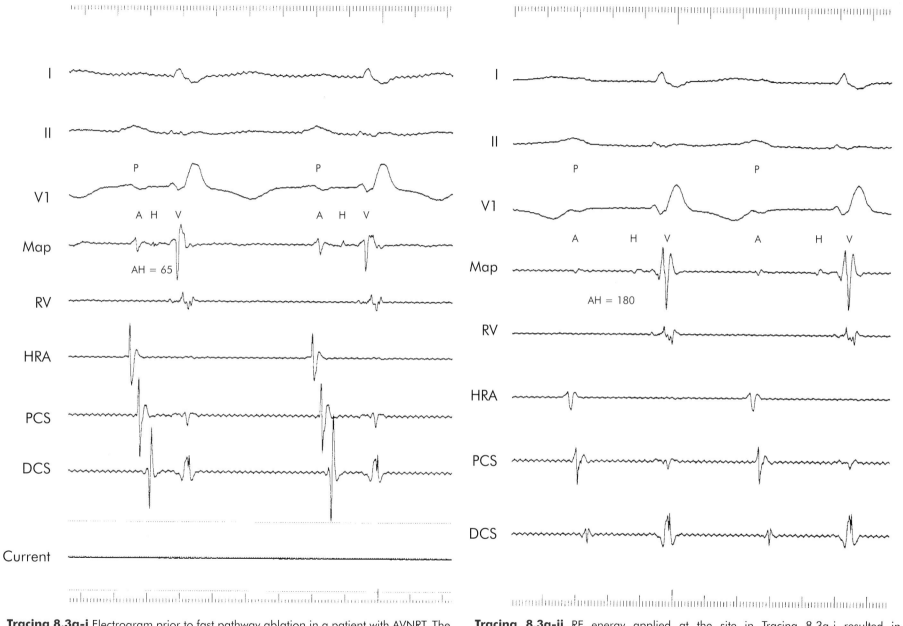

Tracing 8.3a-i Electrogram prior to fast pathway ablation in a patient with AVNRT. The ablation electrogram demonstrates a fairly balanced atrial and ventricular electrogram with a small His deflection.

Tracing 8.3a-ii RF energy applied at the site in Tracing 8.3a-i resulted in prolongation of the AH and PR interval. AVNRT was no longer inducible.

8.3B 'SLOW PATHWAY' ABLATION

The slow pathway usually enters the AV node along Koch's triangle from a posterior (properly, inferior) direction (Figure 8.3b-i). Catheter ablation is directed at tissue in the region between the CS os and the tricuspid annulus, starting at a posterior location, and avoiding sites with a visible His potential. With sufficient perseverance, a dedicated operator can usually identify and target discrete 'slow pathway potentials' (see Section 4.4), but an approach combining the anatomical landmarks and electrogram morphology (a large ventricular electrogram with a small, complex atrial electrogram, often with a 'bump and spike' shape) can be equally successful.

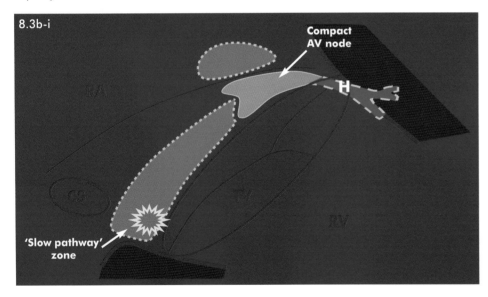

The risk of AV block requiring permanent pacing is around 0.5–1.0% if ablation is performed at or posterior to the level of the CS os. However, to abolish slow pathway conduction it is sometimes necessary to ablate closer to the compact node itself, and the risk of AV block increases progressively with anterior (superior) movement of the ablation site. It is important to discuss this risk thoroughly with the patient before commencing the procedure: the likelihood of success increases with a more aggressive approach, but at the price of a higher risk of damage to the node. Even a 0.5% risk of pacing is quite unacceptable to many young patients, while an older patient with severe symptoms may find this a minor issue.

'Slow pathway' ablation is illustrated in Figure 8.3b-ii, which shows fluoroscopic images in left anterior oblique (LAO) and right anterior oblique (RAO) projections. The ablation catheter (ABL) is positioned slightly anterior and superior to the coronary sinus os, indicated by the PCS electrode. This would be a typical location for successful slow pathway ablation. However, it is our practice to start mapping and ablation at a more inferoposterior location (around the level of the os itself) where there is less risk of damage to the compact AV node. If success is not achieved at this location, ablation can be performed at more anterosuperior sites, but the risk of damage to the node increases progressively.

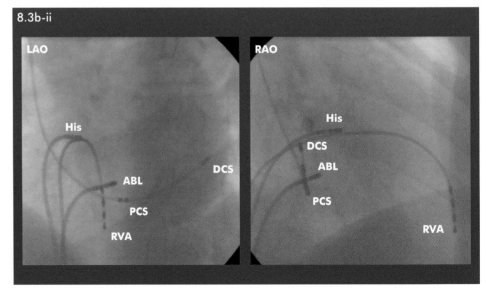

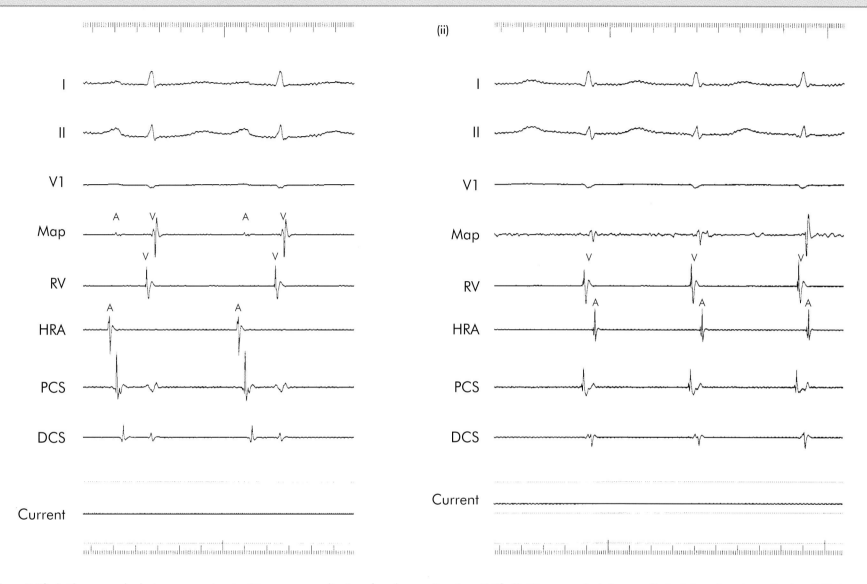

Tracing 8.3b-i The sensed electrogram prior to RF energy application for slow pathway ablation in a patient with AVNRT. Using a combined 'anatomic' and 'electrogram' approach, the catheter has been positioned along the tricuspid annulus slightly anterior to the CS, and advanced to obtain an electrogram with a large ventricular and small atrial deflection (A). There is no His deflection at this location.

Tracing 8.3b-ii RF energy is being applied at the site where Tracing 8.3b-i was recorded. Junctional rhythm with a cycle length of 500 ms is induced by energy application. The A:V ratio is 1:1, suggesting that antegrade conduction through the His-Purkinje system and retrograde conduction to the atria are unaffected by the ablation. This response, which is usually seen within a few seconds of current application, is a marker of a successful location for slow pathway ablation.

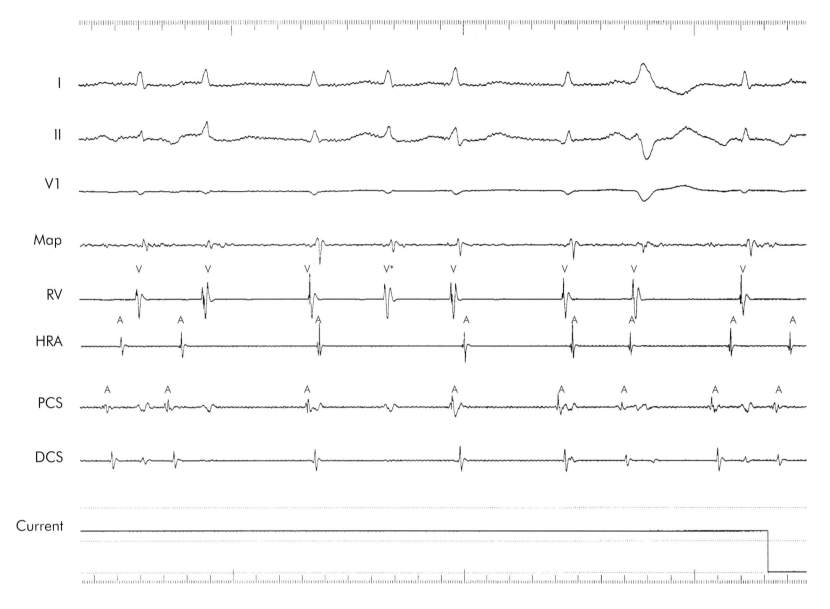

Tracing 8.3b-iii RF energy application at a location midway between the CS orifice and the His recording position. The first two beats represent atrial ectopy, probably arising from irritation by the ablation catheter (atrial activation, earliest at the proximal coronary sinus, precedes ventricular activation). Following this, there is rapid junctional tachycardia with VA block on the second beat (*). This suggests retrograde fast pathway injury, indicating the immediate need to discontinue energy application.

Successful ablation of the slow pathway is accompanied by junctional tachycardia caused by automaticity in the heated tissue. During ablation, the atrial and ventricular electrograms must be watched keenly: ventricular complexes that are not conducted to the atrium suggest fast pathway injury, while non-conducted atrial complexes suggest injury to the node itself, which may become permanent if the current is not immediately discontinued.

8.3C   ENDPOINTS FOR SLOW PATHWAY ABLATION

A variety of endpoints have been suggested for slow pathway ablation. Usually, a clear outcome can be achieved, with abolition of the discontinuity in the AV nodal conduction curve (Figure 8.3c). This is usually accompanied by some degree of shortening of the fast pathway effective refractory period, i.e. AV block occurs at a shorter A1A2 interval after ablation than the interval at which the jump occurred prior to ablation.

Undoubtedly if dual AV nodal physiology, AV nodal echoes and AVNRT are all demonstrated before ablation, and none is seen after, this indicates an ideal result. However, AVNRT and 'echoes' due to reentry in the AV node (see Section 4.2A) are often rendered non-inducible while dual AV nodal physiology persists. If tachycardia is non-inducible even during isoproterenol infusion, it may be appropriate to discontinue the procedure and observe the patient for a period, to assess the clinical impact of ablation. Conducting a repeat procedure in the small number of patients who do have a clinical recurrence is preferable to exposing all patients to the risk of a more aggressive ablation approach that is unnecessary for most.

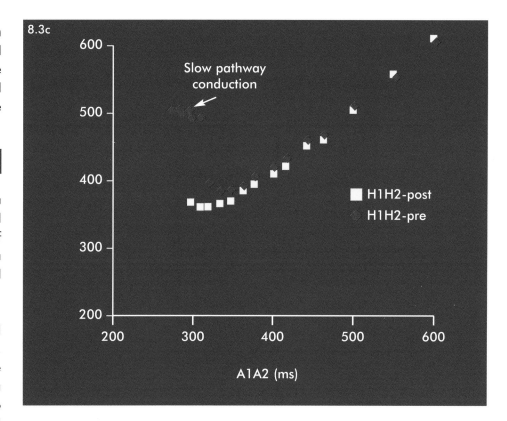

Conventionally, the source of a focal tachycardia or focal ectopy (that is, arising from an automatic focus or micro-reentrant circuit) is identified grossly by examination of the tachycardia morphology. As discussed in Section 3, a superior P-wave axis during atrial tachycardia suggests a low origin for atrial activation, such as the posterior septum, and a rightward axis suggests a left atrial origin. In ventricular tachycardia (VT) (see Section 7), the QRS morphology and axis can give similar clues to origin. More accurate localization is obtained using catheter mapping techniques.

8.4A PACE-MAPPING

The location of the focus can be more closely approximated by comparing the P-wave or QRS morphology during tachycardia to that elicited by pacing from the exploring catheter – pace-mapping (Figure 8.4a). As the catheter moves closer to the focus, the pace-map obtained approximates the spontaneous morphology more closely. However, proximity to the focus cannot be inferred until the paced ECG resembles the tachycardia ECG in all 12 leads. Because details of QRS morphology are more easily distinguished than those of P-wave morphology, pace-mapping is more useful in ventricular than atrial tachycardias.

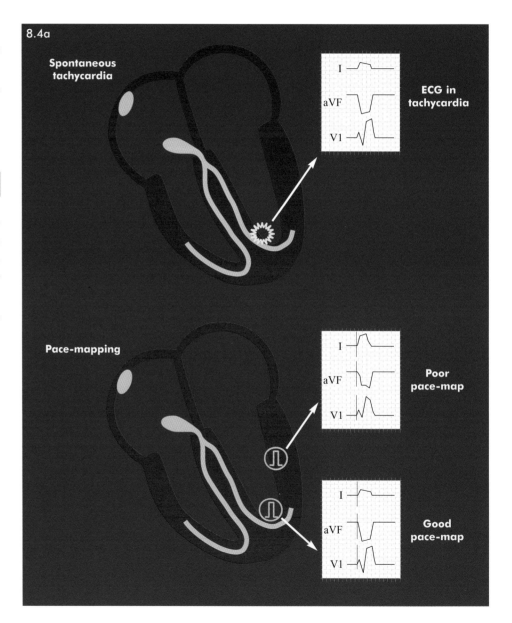

8.4a

Spontaneous tachycardia

ECG in tachycardia

Pace-mapping

Poor pace-map

Good pace-map

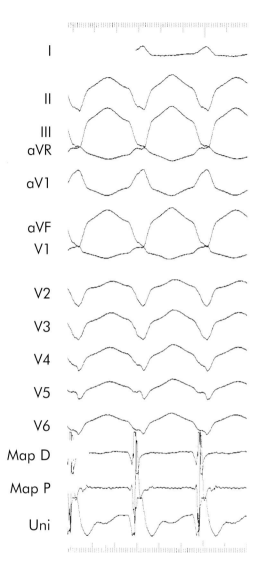
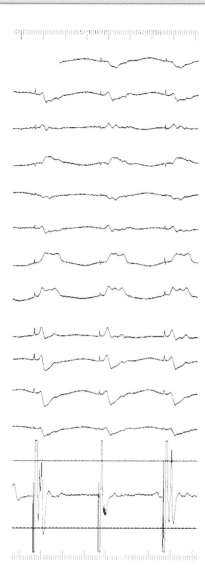
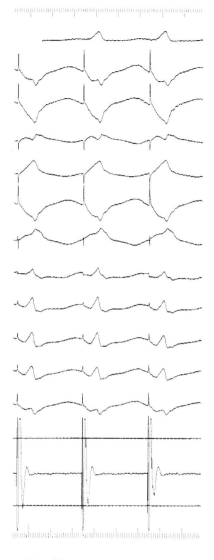

Lead labels (left column): I, II, III, aVR, aV1, aVF, V1, V2, V3, V4, V5, V6, Map D, Map P, Uni

Tracing 8.4a-i Pace-mapping in a patient with idiopathic VT arising from the apical interventricular septum. The spontaneous tachycardia is seen in 12 ECG leads and the ablation catheter (Map D = distal bipole, Map P = proximal bipole, Uni = unipolar electrogram).

Tracing 8.4a-ii The next panel shows pacing from the distal electrode pair of the ablation catheter. The paced QRS morphology does not resemble the spontaneous tachycardia morphology, suggesting that the catheter is far removed from the origin of VT.

Tracing 8.4a-iii As the ablation/pacing catheter is advanced towards the apical septum, the limb leads begin to resemble the spontaneous tachycardia morphology, but the precordial leads remain a poor match.

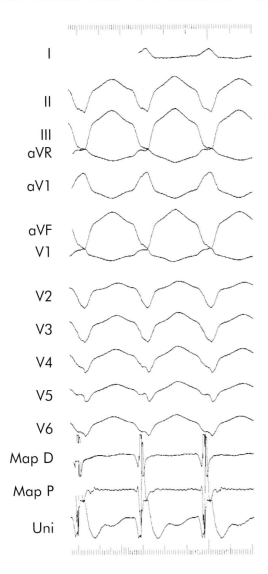

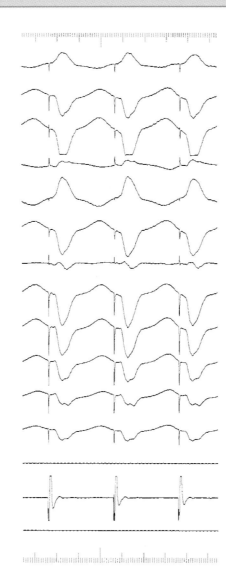

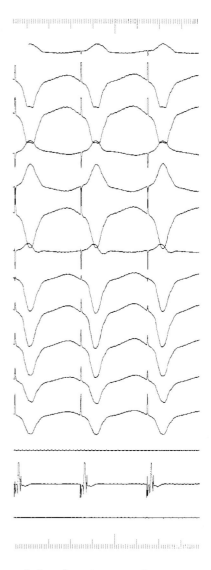

Tracing 8.4a-iv The spontaneous tachycardia shown again for comparison.

Tracing 8.4a-v After repositioning of the ablation/pacing catheter, a fair match is obtained in 11 of 12 leads. The mismatch is most noticeable in V1, which is isoelectric during pacing, but strongly positive in tachycardia.

Tracing 8.4a-vi Minor adjustment of the ablation/pacing catheter resulted in a reasonable (albeit not perfect) match in 12 of 12 leads, with a largely positive deflection in V1. This suggests very close proximity to the tachycardia focus.

8.4B   ACTIVATION MAPPING

Pace-mapping is a useful technique for 'homing in' on the region of interest, as it does not require continuous tachycardia, which may be difficult to sustain or poorly tolerated. However, activation mapping is usually required to pinpoint the focus accurately. During tachycardia, the mapping catheter explores the endocardium to identify the site where the earliest electrogram relative to a fixed reference is recorded. This reference point is generally taken from the surface ECG (the onset of the P-wave or QRS complex), but a distant endocardial electrogram may be used instead. A suitable site for ablation is (i) one at which local electrogram precedes any other evidence of activity (other endocardial electrograms or surface ECG), (ii) one from which any movement results in a later electrogram, and (iii) one at which the unipolar electrogram shows a sharp initial negative deflection. A shortcoming of activation mapping is that catheter-induced ectopy can satisfy these criteria and cause confusion, especially in the mapping of non-sustained tachycardia.

Figure 8.4b shows idealized electrograms from mapping catheters simultaneously recording at three sites in the region of a tachycardia focus. At site C, the electrogram onset is equal in timing to the reference (surface ECG). The proximal bipole (3–4) is equal in timing to the distal bipole (1–2). The unipolar electrogram shows a shallow, slurred 'QS' morphology – this 'cavity potential' reflects activation over the whole chamber with rather poor contact. At site B, the bipolar electrograms are both earlier than the reference, so this site is closer to the focus than site C. Proximity is also indicated by the sharp unipolar electrogram. However, the latter begins with a small positive deflection, indicating that endocardial activation initially travels toward the electrode from the focus. The location could therefore be improved on. At site A, the bipolar electrograms are earlier still, and the distal bipole is clearly earlier than both the proximal bipole and the reference. The unipolar electrogram commences with a sharp negative deflection, indicating that all endocardial activation is traveling away from the electrode, i.e. activation commences directly beneath the electrode.

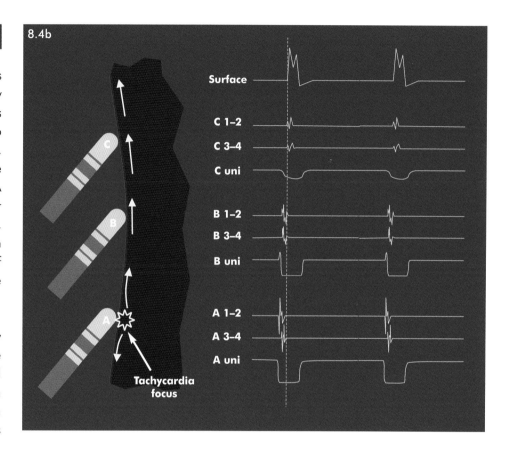

8.4b

Surface
C 1–2
C 3–4
C uni
B 1–2
B 3–4
B uni
A 1–2
A 3–4
A uni

Tachycardia focus

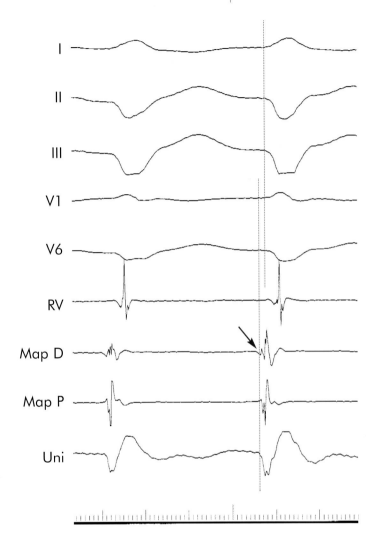

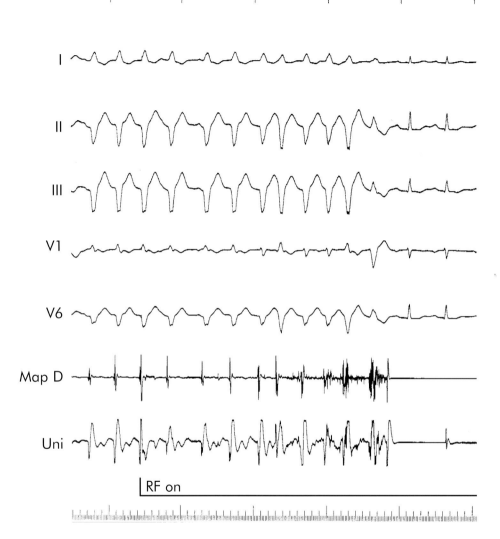

Tracing 8.4b-i Electrogram recorded during spontaneous tachycardia at the site shown in Tracing 8.4a-vi. Note that the bipolar electrogram (arrowed) precedes the QRS onset by ~20 ms, and that the unipolar electrogram shows a sharp negative initial deflection. These findings indicate that the catheter is at or near the 'exit' site from which ventricular activation spreads.

Tracing 8.4b-ii Successful ablation of the septal ventricular tachycardia at the site shown in Tracings 8.4a-vi and b-i. During tachycardia, RF energy is applied. There is immediate irregular acceleration of the tachycardia, followed by termination after 3.4 s of current application. Subsequent to the completion of a 60 s current application at this site, tachycardia could no longer be induced.

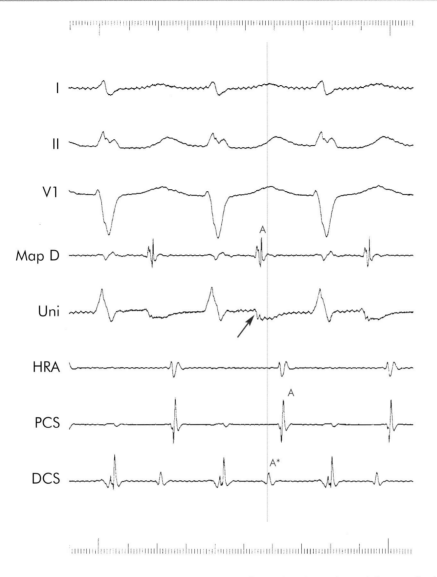

Tracing 8.4b-iii Activation mapping of an ectopic left atrial tachycardia. Of the standard electrode positions, the distal coronary sinus records the earliest atrial electrogram (A*) and is used as the reference. The ablation catheter (Map D) is positioned 1 cm above the posterolateral mitral annulus where it records a sharp atrial electrogram with a far-field ventricular electrogram. The unipolar electrogram (Uni) has a sharp negative atrial deflection (arrowed). Ablation at this site resulted in acceleration followed by termination of the atrial tachycardia.

Accessory AV pathways are located using similar principles to those described above. For patients with overt pre-excitation (delta waves), a number of algorithms have been described that identify the approximate region of interest, based on QRS morphology in sinus rhythm. Further clues to pathway location are obtained from the diagnostic study, as described in Section 6. The mitral or tricuspid annulus is then explored with a steerable catheter, using activation mapping to locate the pathway precisely.

8.5A ANATOMY OF ACCESSORY PATHWAYS

The exact anatomy of accessory pathways is variable (Figure 8.5a). Most are fine strands of myocardial tissue bridging the AV valve annulus near the endocardium, but some are intimately related to the vessels in the AV groove (especially venous structures near the CS os), and epicardial bands of tissue are occasionally seen. At least 10% of patients have multiple pathways. The figure shows common relationships between accessory pathways and structures in the left AV groove.

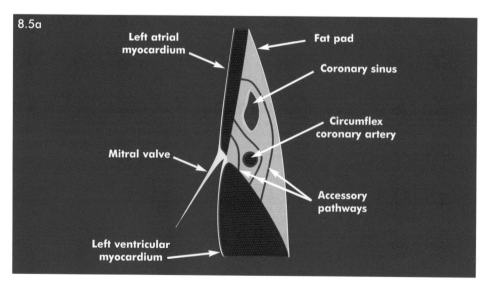

8.5B CATHETER TECHNIQUE

For right-sided and septal accessory pathways, the tricuspid annulus is mapped using a catheter introduced from the right femoral vein. The annulus is almost always mapped from the atrial aspect of the valve, as access from the ventricular aspect is extremely difficult. Stable catheter positions can usually be achieved at septal and posterior locations. Mapping and ablation of the less common right free wall accessory pathways can be technically more challenging because of catheter instability. However, an approach via the superior vena cava or using one of a variety of preshaped sheaths can improve stability.

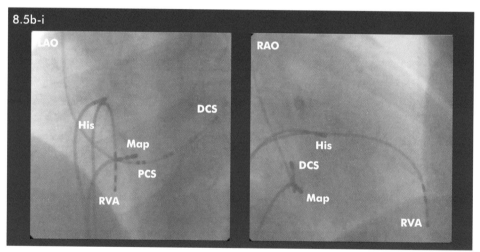

Figure 8.5b-i illustrates catheter mapping of a right posteroseptal accessory pathway (infero-paraseptal in the proposed new nomenclature, see Section 5.3), showing fluoroscopic images in left anterior oblique (LAO) and right anterior oblique (RAO) projections. The proximal pole of the coronary sinus catheter (PCS) is positioned in the CS os. The mapping catheter (Map) is positioned on the tricuspid annulus just in front of the os.

Two approaches can be taken to map the mitral annulus and ablate left-sided accessory pathways: the retrograde approach is via the femoral artery and across the aortic valve to the left ventricle. Using this retrograde approach, the mitral annulus can be mapped either from below (Figure 8.5b-ii, left) or (through the valve) from above. The alternative approach to the mitral annulus is to gain access to the left atrium using a sheath advanced through a trans-septal puncture (or, if present, a patent foramen ovale). With the trans-septal approach, most of the mitral annulus is easily explored from above (Figure 8.5b-ii, right), but catheter stability can occasionally be difficult to achieve in some locations. Again, a variety of preshaped sheaths are available to help this task. Each approach to the left side carries specific risks. With the trans-septal approach, there is a risk of cardiac perforation and tamponade; with the retrograde approach, the risk is of damage to the proximal coronary arteries, the aortic valve and the submitral apparatus. These risks can be minimized by appropriate training, careful technique and instant recognition of an incorrect catheter position. With either technique, it is usual to heparinize the patient once access to the left side of the heart has been gained and an endocavitary location has been confirmed by the recording of left atrial and ventricular electrograms.

Figure 8.5b-iii illustrates catheter mapping of a left free wall accessory pathway via a trans-septal approach, showing fluoroscopic images in LAO and RAO projections. The mapping catheter crosses the interatrial septum (TS), curves within the left atrium, and is mapping the mitral annulus at a point between the second and third bipoles of the coronary sinus catheter.

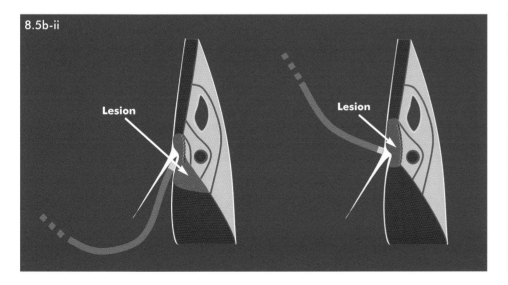

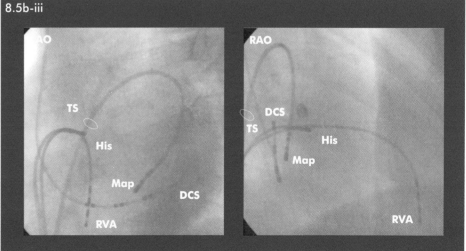

8.5C   MAPPING ANTEGRADE CONDUCTION OVER AN ACCESSORY PATHWAY

Pathways that conduct antegradely can be mapped during sinus rhythm. The principle is to find the location on the mitral or tricuspid annulus where ventricular activation is earliest. Commonly, the ventricle is activated partially by the AV node and partially by the pathway, which can cause difficulty with mapping, especially if the pathway is near the node (septal locations). This fusion between activation over the pathway and the AV node can be reduced by pacing the atrium at a rate sufficient to cause delay in the AV node and thus maximize pre-excitation (Figure 8.5c), or by pacing at a location nearer the pathway than the node (e.g. the coronary sinus for a left-sided or posteroseptal pathway – see Section 5.5). Ventricular activation is then almost exclusively over the pathway.

Using one of the approaches described above, the ablation catheter explores the annulus while the following electrogram characteristics are sought. Firstly, good tissue contact and a location on the annulus are confirmed by the presence of sharp electrograms from both atrium and ventricle. Secondly, the location on the annulus closest to the ventricular insertion of the pathway is sought using the same principles as in Figure 8.4b. The electrogram should be at least as early as the onset of the surface delta wave, and is usually earlier. Movement along the annulus in either direction from this location results in a later ventricular electrogram. Finally, if the unipolar electrogram is examined, it should begin with a sharp negative deflection. Near the accessory pathway location, the atrial and ventricular components of the electrogram can be so close that they are hard to distinguish.

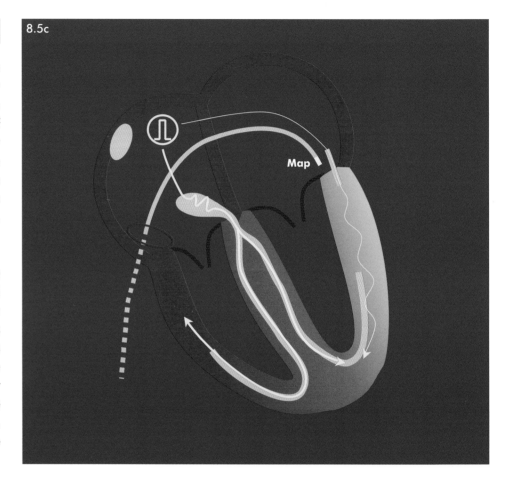

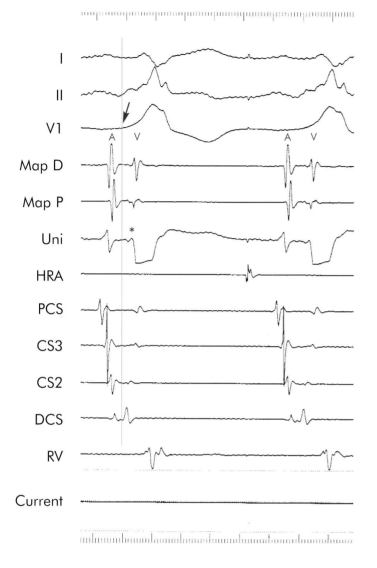

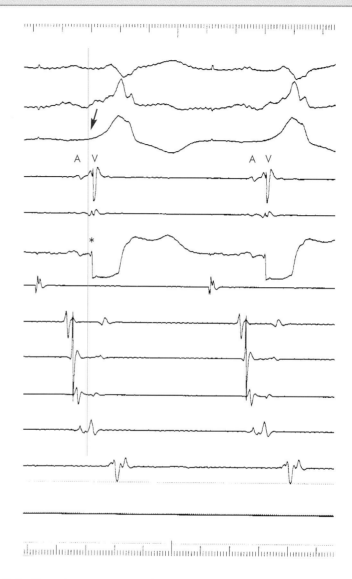

Tracing 8.5c-i Mapping during atrial pacing in a patient with a left lateral accessory pathway. The distal ablation electrogram (Map D) records atrial and ventricular electrograms that are both sharp, indicating a position on the annulus. However, the ventricular component is at least 30 ms later than the earliest ventricular activation, seen on both the surface ECG (arrow and dashed reference line) and the low amplitude early ventricular component of the unipolar electrogram (asterisked). This location is therefore some distance from the accessory pathway and is unlikely to be a successful ablation site.

Tracing 8.5c-ii Further mapping in the same patient records an earlier ventricular electrogram, now approximately 10 ms after the reference. The unipolar electrogram has a small, sharp, initial positive deflection (R-wave, asterisked), suggesting that the catheter is close to, but not yet at, the site of earliest ventricular activation.

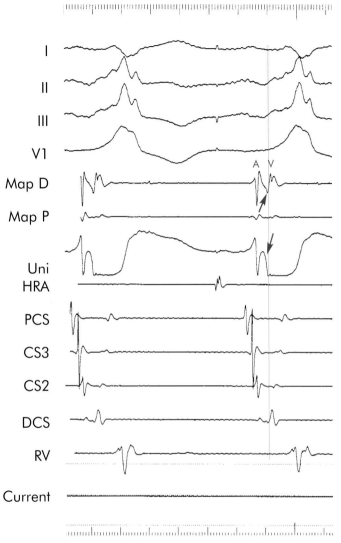

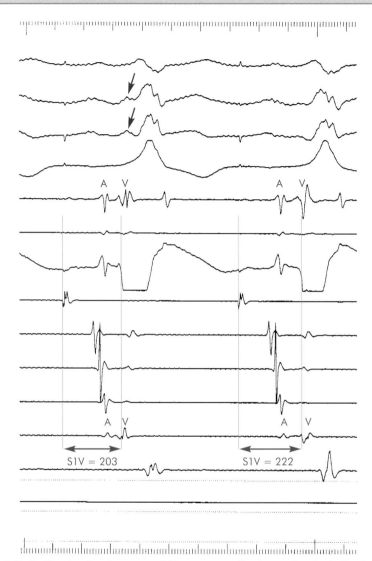

Tracing 8.5c-iii Further mapping in the same patient records an earlier ventricular electrogram (arrowed on the bipolar and unipolar electrograms), now just preceding the delta wave by 10 ms. Note that there is near fusion of the bipolar atrial and ventricular electrograms, with a sharply negative unipolar electrogram (Q wave).

Tracing 8.5c-iv Shortly after the onset of RF energy application at the site in Tracing 8.5c-iii, block occurs in the accessory pathway. The pattern of pre-excitation on the surface ECG changes (note the disappearance of the initial positive deflection in leads II and III, arrowed), the local AV interval at the mapping electrode increases, and the ventricular activation sequence in the coronary sinus leads changes, with a 19 ms increase in the stimulus-V interval in the DCS. However, pre-excitation on the surface ECG is not abolished, and the left ventricular electrograms (from the CS and mapping catheter) are still very early. These findings suggest the presence of a second left-sided accessory pathway. RF current was continued at this site for a full 60 s to complete elimination of the first accessory pathway, before attention was turned to mapping of the second pathway.

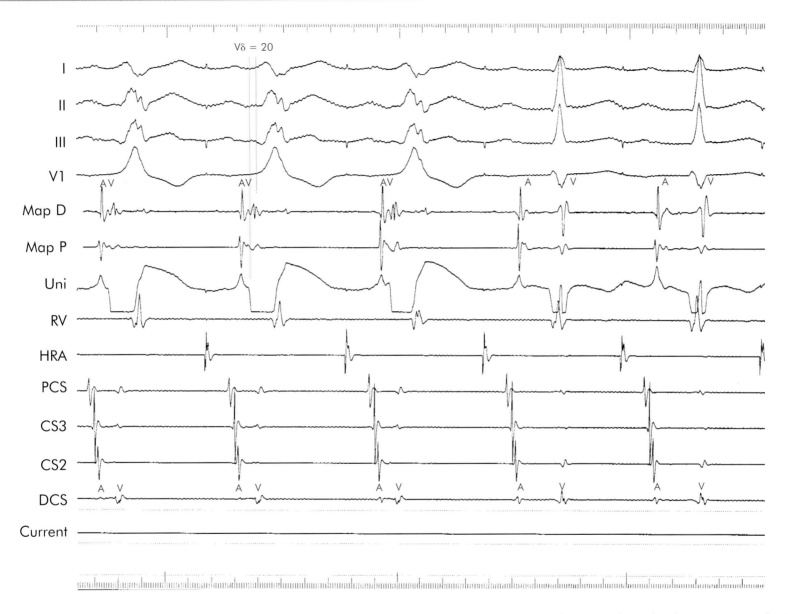

Tracing 8.5c-v The second accessory pathway has been mapped to a more proximal location on the mitral annulus. The tracing shows the electrograms just after the onset of RF current. On the first three beats, the local atrial and ventricular electrograms are nearly fused, the ventricular electrogram precedes the delta wave by 20 ms, and the unipolar electrogram has a sharp initial negative deflection. After the third beat on the tracing, block occurs in the second accessory pathway: pre-excitation on the surface ECG abruptly disappears and the AV interval increases both on the local ablation electrogram and in the CS leads.

8.5D   MAPPING RETROGRADE CONDUCTION OVER AN ACCESSORY PATHWAY

Mapping and ablation of an accessory pathway can also be performed during retrograde conduction. In this case, the aim is to locate the atrial insertion of the pathway by seeking the earliest atrial electrogram. The same principles apply as with mapping during antegrade conduction: a signal showing both atrial and ventricular electrograms indicates a position on the annulus, and the location giving the earliest atrial electrogram is sought. If mapping is performed during ventricular pacing, conduction may occur over both the AV node and the pathway, which may confuse the picture. As with antegrade mapping, this problem can be helped by pacing at a higher rate (Figure 8.5d), or near the pathway (e.g. left ventricular basal pacing for a left-sided pathway), to favor conduction over the pathway.

Mapping can also be performed during orthodromic AV reentrant tachycardia (AVRT), which guarantees that atrial activation is solely over the pathway. The sudden change in rhythm and rate that occurs when ablation is performed during tachycardia may displace the ablation catheter from the successful site. This can be minimized by ventricular pacing slightly faster than the rate of AVRT (entrainment) during current application.

It should be noted that the optimal sites on the mitral or tricuspid annulus may differ when mapping antegradely and retrogradely, as many pathways are 'oblique', i.e. their atrial and ventricular insertions are some way apart on the annulus.

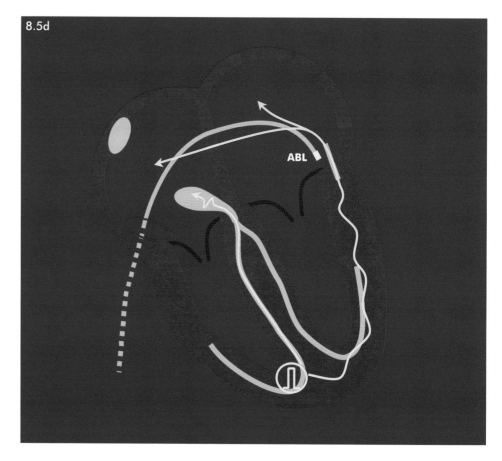

8.5d

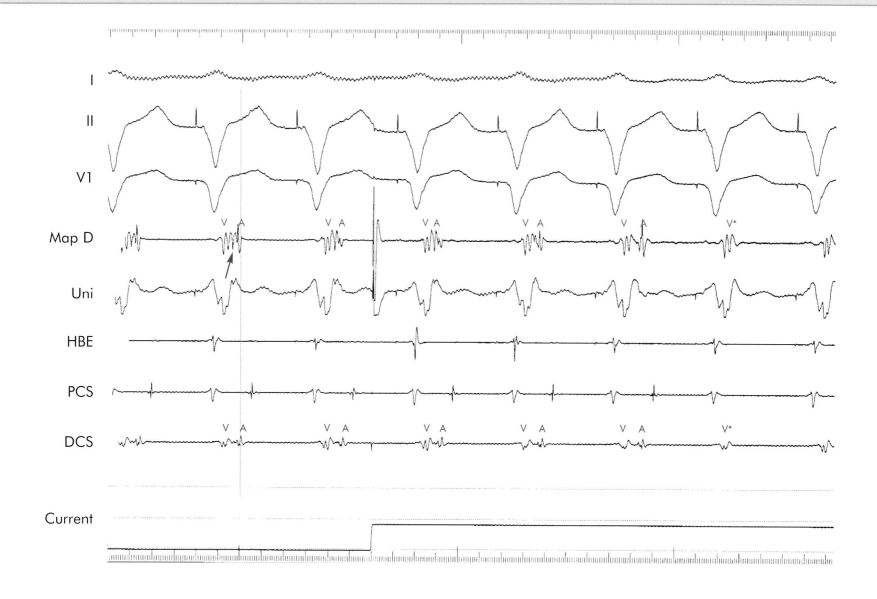

Tracing 8.5d-i Ablation of a concealed left lateral accessory pathway during ventricular pacing at cycle length (CL) 500 ms. The ablation catheter (Map D) records a balanced atrial and ventricular electrogram, with atrial activation earlier than the reference (dashed line) taken from the atrial electrogram at the distal CS. The sharp deflection between the ventricular and atrial electrograms might be an accessory pathway potential (arrowed). VA block indicating successful ablation occurs 1.6 s after the onset of current (V*).

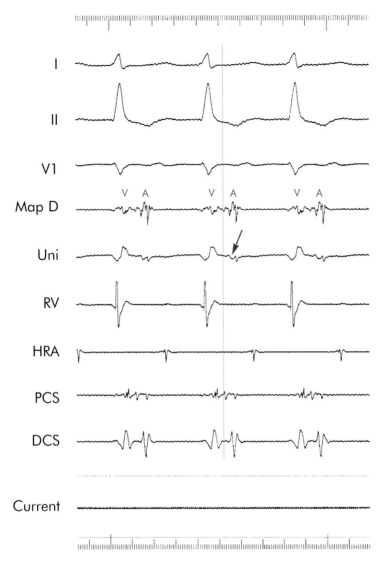

Tracing 8.5d-ii Mapping of a concealed posteroseptal accessory pathway during orthodromic AVRT. The sensed electrogram on the ablation catheter (Map D) is complex, and the short VA interval suggests proximity to the pathway. However, the atrial electrogram is later than the reference (cursor) taken from the proximal coronary sinus, a small positive unipolar atrial deflection is seen (arrow), and the ventricular electrogram is of very low amplitude. For these reasons, catheter ablation at this site is unlikely to be successful.

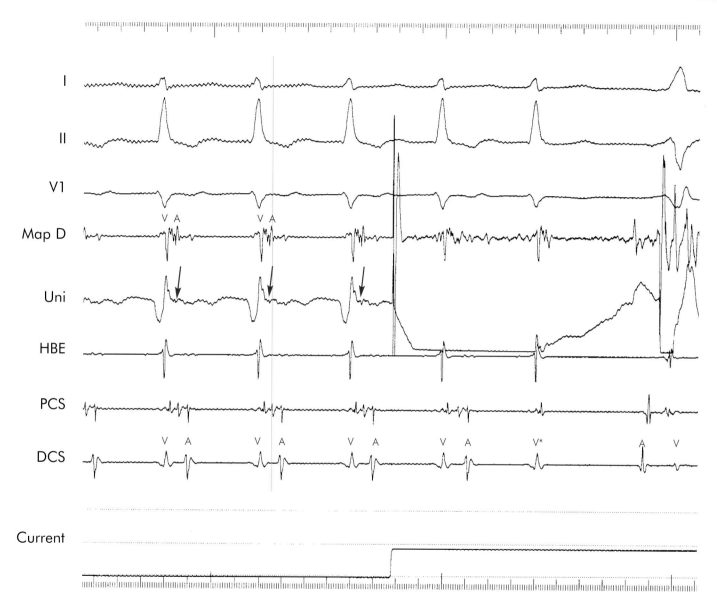

Tracing 8.5d-iii The catheter has been repositioned. There is now a larger ventricular deflection and continuous electrical activity with very early atrial activation, now preceding the reference electrogram (cursor). The small unipolar atrial deflection is negative (arrows). There may be an accessory pathway potential between the ventricular and atrial electrograms seen in map D. 700 ms after the onset of RF current, AVRT terminates due to block in the pathway (the last event in tachycardia is a ventricular electrogram – V*).

Accessory pathway (AP) potentials may be encountered during mapping and used to localize and ablate pathways. These potentials are characteristically of low amplitude but high frequency, and are detected between the atrial and ventricular electrogram. They represent direct registration of accessory pathway activation, analogous to His bundle potentials. They can be detected in sinus rhythm, during atrial or ventricular pacing, or during tachycardia. Their presence is often suspected when there is 'continuous' electrical activity between the atrial and ventricular electrograms. Accessory pathway potentials can be distinguished from fractionated local electrograms by observing the responses to atrial and ventricular extrastimuli.

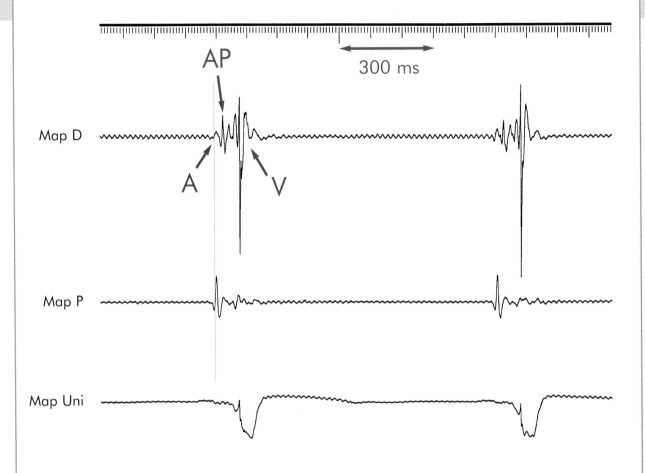

Tracing 8.5e An accessory pathway potential recorded during an ablation procedure. The apparently continuous electrical activity in the distal mapping bipole (Map D) can be separated into a small atrial component (corresponding to the atrial electrogram on the proximal bipole), the AP potential and the ventricular electrogram. This appearance is highly predictive of a successful ablation site.

8.6A   ISTHMUS ABLATION FOR TYPICAL ATRIAL FLUTTER

The tachycardias discussed above can be abolished by ablation of a very small area of tissue critical to the circuit (a focus, the AV nodal 'slow pathway', an accessory AV pathway). In contrast, abolition of other macro-reentrant circuits requires the creation of a line of block across the path of the circuit. In typical atrial flutter, the circuit passes through an anatomically-defined channel – the isthmus between the inferior vena cava and the tricuspid annulus. This isthmus offers a number of advantages as a target for ablation. Firstly, it is an obligatory route for the circuit – the flutter wavefront cannot find an alternative path if conduction through the isthmus is blocked. Secondly, it is a relatively safe area to ablate, with a low risk of damage to the AV node or perforation of the right atrial free wall. Finally, interruption of conduction across the isthmus usually involves creation of a line of block of limited length (usually only 2–3 cm).

To create a line of isthmus block (dotted blue line), the ablation catheter is advanced from the femoral vein into the right atrium and across the tricuspid valve (Figure 8.6a-i). The line is commenced at a point on the ventricular side of the tricuspid annulus (i.e. where a ventricular electrogram is seen, but the atrial electrogram just disappears). A series of lesions is created as the catheter is gradually withdrawn to the atrial side of the annulus, then back toward the inferior vena cava (IVC), where an electrogram is no longer visible. As long as it is continuous, the exact location of the line is not critical: success can be achieved posteriorly (6 o'clock or beyond on the tricuspid annulus in the LAO view) or anteriorly toward the CS os. The choice of location is generally determined by practical considerations, which influence the ease with which a line of block can be created. The ridges of pectinate muscle that straddle the isthmus make the endocardial surface irregular, impeding electrode contact in places, and where the tissue is particularly thick it can be difficult to create a transmural lesion using a conventional catheter. It is helpful to perform a 'dry run' along the proposed line, without delivering energy, as this gives some idea regarding catheter stability and the surface irregularity.

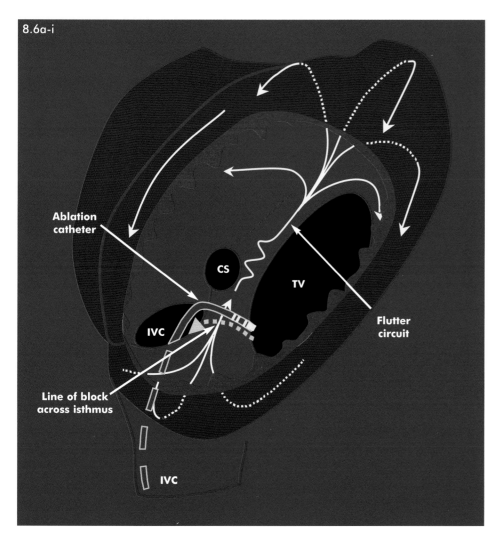

8.6a-i

Ablation catheter

Line of block across isthmus

CS

TV

IVC

IVC

Flutter circuit

It has been found that the best predictor of success with an isthmus ablation is not just that atrial flutter is rendered non-inducible, but that conduction block in both directions across the isthmus is created. If bidirectional block is achieved (which is possible in most cases), recurrence of typical flutter is very rare. However, the procedure does not prevent atrial fibrillation (which often coexists) from recurring.

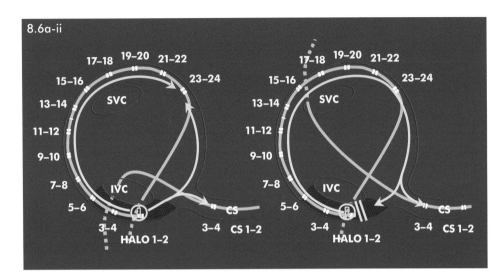

8.6a-ii

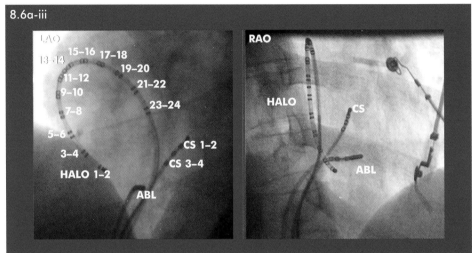

8.6a-iii

Figure 8.6a-ii illustrates atrial activation during low right atrial pacing, before (left) and after (right) creation of a line of block across the isthmus. A multipolar catheter has been placed along the crista terminalis, parallel to the tricuspid annulus, with its distal pole (HALO 1–2) in the low right atrium and its proximal pole (23–24) at the roof of the septum, not far from the bundle of His. Another electrode records coronary sinus activation. Prior to ablation, activation spreads from the low right atrial pacing site in both directions, and reaches the proximal CS fairly rapidly across the isthmus. After ablation, counterclockwise propagation across the isthmus is blocked, so the coronary sinus is reached later, by clockwise propagation all the way round the tricuspid annulus.

Figure 8.6a-iii illustrates placement of catheters for ablation of the subeustachian isthmus. A 24-pole catheter is deployed along the crista terminalis, a quadripolar catheter in the proximal segment of the coronary sinus, and an 8-mm tip ablation catheter is at the isthmus itself. Left: left anterior oblique view; right: right anterior oblique view.

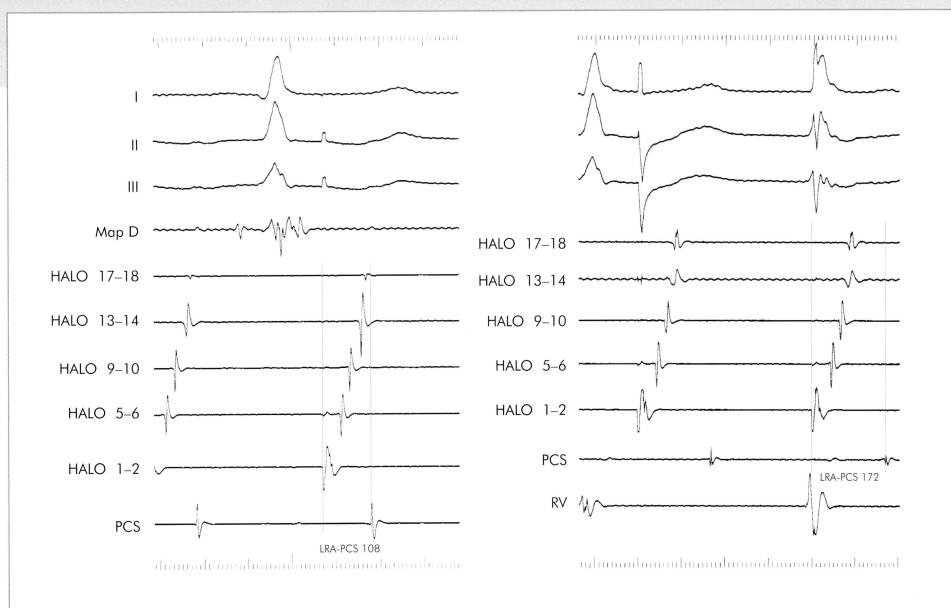

Tracing 8.6a-ii Atrial activation during pacing from the low right atrium before (left) and after (right) isthmus ablation for atrial flutter. The electrodes are labeled as in Figure 8.6a-ii (for clarity, only a selection of the HALO bipoles are displayed). After ablation, atrial activation along the multipolar catheter is unchanged, but CS (CS 5–6) activation is delayed by 64 ms, indicating counterclockwise block in the isthmus.

Figure 8.6a-iv illustrates atrial activation during coronary sinus (CS) pacing before (left) and after (right) creation of a line of block across the isthmus. Before ablation, activation spreads round the tricuspid annulus in both clockwise and counterclockwise directions, with the lateral right atrium depolarized last. After ablation, depolarization can no longer reach the low right atrium directly across the isthmus, so activation is entirely counterclockwise.

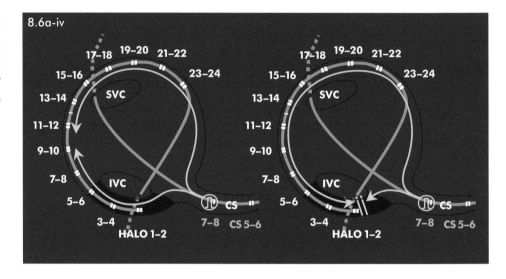

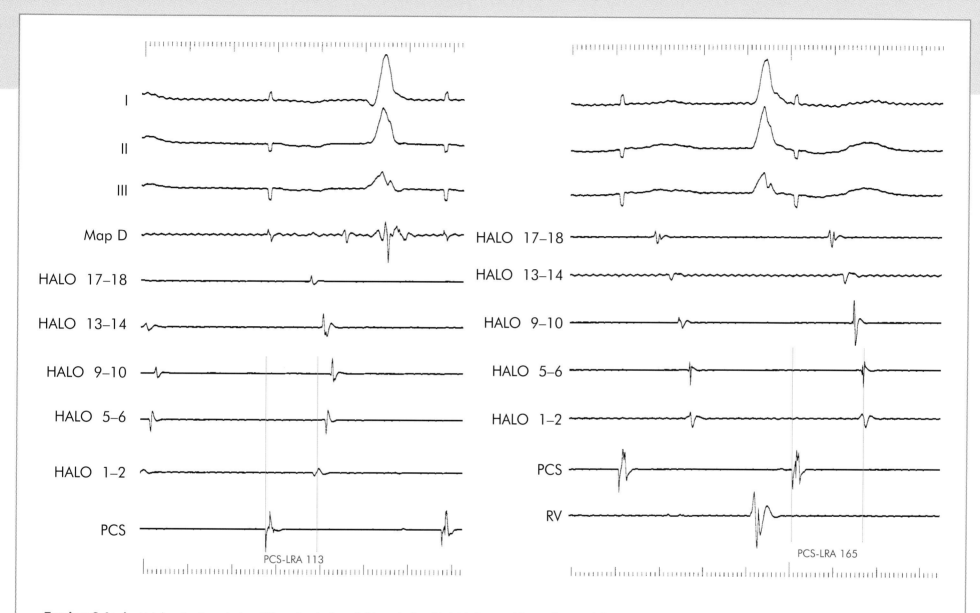

Tracing 8.6a-iv Atrial activation during CS pacing before (left) and after (right) isthmus ablation for atrial flutter. The electrodes on the multipolar catheter are labeled as in Figure 8.6a-iv (for clarity, only a selection of the HALO bipoles are displayed). Prior to ablation, there is simultaneous clockwise and counterclockwise activation around the tricuspid annulus, with the lateral right atrium (HALO 9–10) depolarized last. Following isthmus block, activation of the distal pole in the low lateral right atrium (HALO 1–2) is delayed by 52 ms, and activation of poles 1–9 is reversed, as the impulse can only propagate in a counterclockwise direction. This indicates clockwise block in the isthmus.

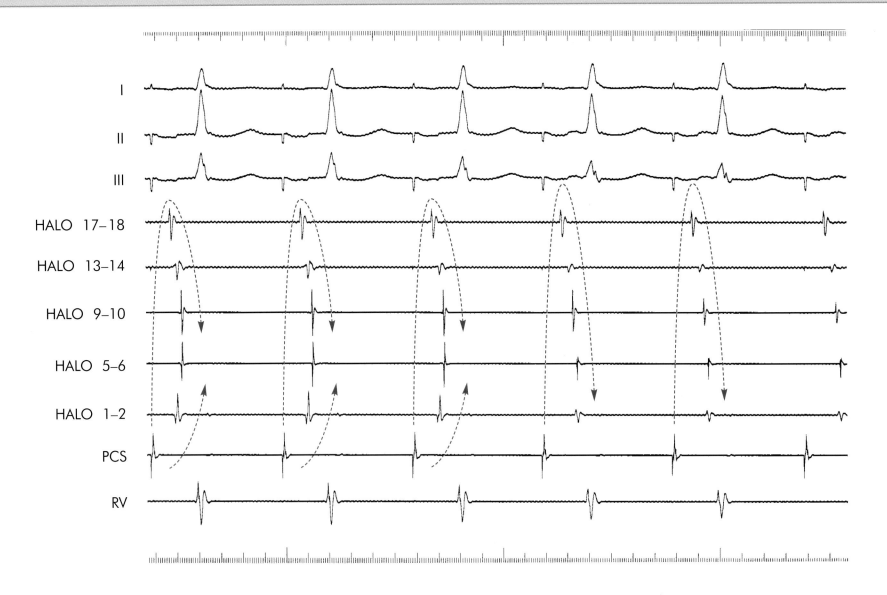

Tracing 8.6a-v In practice, it is common to perform isthmus ablation during CS pacing, as this provides an immediate indication that success may have been achieved, avoiding unnecessary further lesions. This tracing was recorded during the 8th RF application, which completed a line of block across the isthmus. After the first three beats, there is an obvious change in activation, as clockwise block occurs in the isthmus (equivalent to the 'before and after' views in Tracing 8.6a-ii). This suggests that the line of ablation may be complete, but low right pacing is still needed to determine whether the block is bidirectional.

8.6B OTHER MACRO-REENTRANT CIRCUITS

A similar approach can be taken in ablating other macro-reentrant circuits, such as atrial flutter related to a surgical scar (Figure 8.6b). It is often possible to identify the scar by electrogram characteristics and create a line of block between it and another fixed obstacle, such as the inferior vena cava. While this approach is often successful, in most cases of atypical atrial flutter and ventricular tachycardia, mapping and entrainment techniques are needed to define the pathway of the circuit.

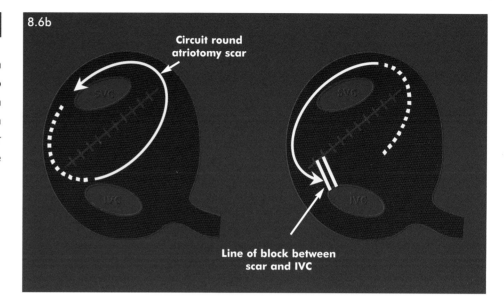

8.6b

Circuit round atriotomy scar

Line of block between scar and IVC

Most macro-reentrant circuits within the atrium or ventricle do not follow paths defined by standard anatomy (typical atrial flutter and bundle branch reentry being exceptions). Some form of mapping is necessary to identify the circuit and the components of its substrate. The purpose in mapping such tachycardias is to find an isthmus of tissue that is an obligatory part of the circuit, and which is small enough to be a reasonable target for ablation. We will confine most of the following discussion to ventricular tachycardia (VT) arising in peri-infarct tissue (scar-related VT).

8.7A   MAPPING AND CATHETER ABLATION FOR SCAR-RELATED VENTRICULAR TACHYCARDIA

Conventional mapping of VT requires the tachycardia to be fairly stable both electrically (i.e. monomorphic tachycardia) and hemodynamically. The best target for ablation has usually been found to be within a zone of slow conduction, generally near its exit point. However, the nature of scar-related VT is such that the substrate may exist for more than one circuit, each of which may have more than one exit point. An extensive procedure may therefore be necessary to eliminate all possible tachycardia circuits in a patient. Only a minority of patients are able to sustain and tolerate VT for a sufficient time to allow the necessary mapping, and this is the principal limitation of conventional mapping methods in this condition.

To reduce the length of time spent mapping tachycardia, a number of preliminary techniques can be used to identify the approximate location of the circuit (Figure 8.7a-i). The QRS morphology and axis on the 12-lead ECG during tachycardia can give a first clue to the location of the reentrant circuit, as described in Section 7.

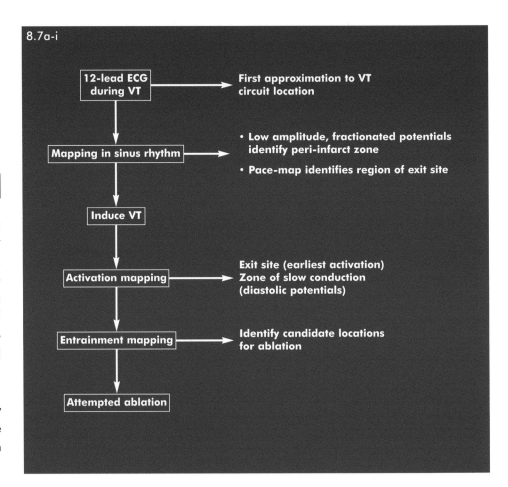

8.7a-i

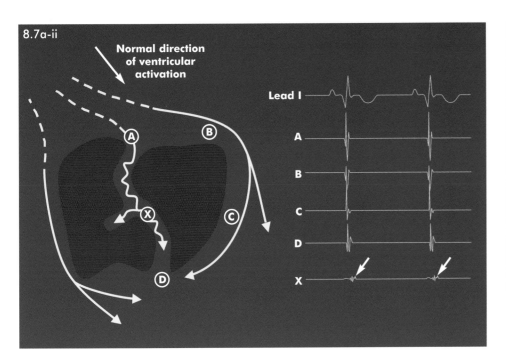

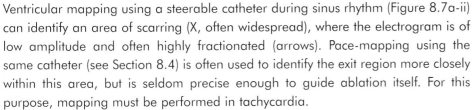

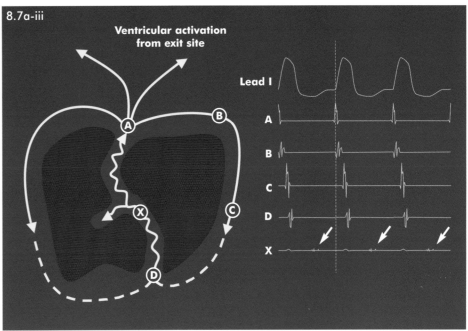

Ventricular mapping using a steerable catheter during sinus rhythm (Figure 8.7a-ii) can identify an area of scarring (X, often widespread), where the electrogram is of low amplitude and often highly fractionated (arrows). Pace-mapping using the same catheter (see Section 8.4) is often used to identify the exit region more closely within this area, but is seldom precise enough to guide ablation itself. For this purpose, mapping must be performed in tachycardia.

Activation mapping (see Section 8.4) during tachycardia can in theory be used to build up a picture of the whole VT circuit, if it is all accessible to an endocardial catheter (Figure 8.7a-iii). However, this is neither necessary nor usually possible: the principal interest is to identify the 'diastolic' inner part of the circuit (D→X→A). This inner part is also known as the 'zone of slow conduction', although the speed is highly variable. The exit point, at which activation emerges from this zone (A), can be mapped like a focal tachycardia or accessory pathway: it is the point at which the earliest sharp ventricular electrogram is recorded. Locations within the zone of slow conduction can be identified from the electrogram during tachycardia: a low amplitude, fractionated potential (arrows) is recorded. Whereas this fractionated electrogram coincides with the QRS complex during sinus rhythm (Figure 8.7a-ii), during tachycardia these potentials are diastolic, as they represent the 'hidden' return limb of the circuit.

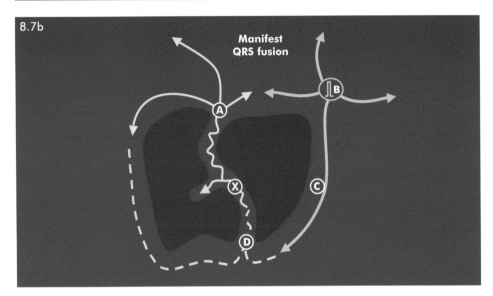

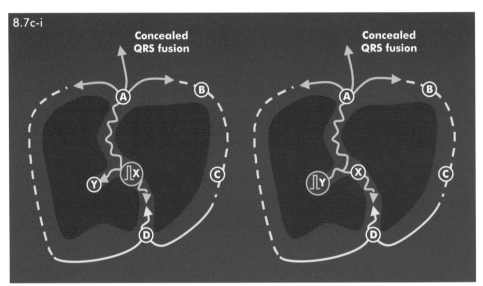

In order to confirm that a promising location is indeed part of the tachycardia circuit, and to determine whether it is likely to be a successful ablation site, it is necessary to attempt entrainment of the tachycardia using the mapping catheter. In addition to the basic principles of entrainment (reviewed in Section 3.4), two further concepts must be understood.

Entrainment of a tachycardia (see Section 3.4) proves that it is due to a reentrant circuit, but not that the pacing site is actually within the circuit. If the excitable gap is large, entrainment can often be achieved by pacing at some distance. In classical entrainment of VT (Figure 8.7b), the ventricle is activated in part from the exit site of the tachycardia (A) and in part directly from the site of pacing (B). The QRS morphology is therefore a fusion between that of the spontaneous tachycardia and that seen in a purely paced rhythm from the same site – entrainment with manifest fusion.

Entrainment from certain sites (X, Y), however, does not allow escape of activation in any direction other than that of the tachycardia circuit. This is because propagation is confined between areas of block, and antidromic propagation is stopped by collision with the preceding orthodromic wavefront. The QRS morphology is therefore identical to that of the tachycardia – entrainment with concealed fusion (Figure 8.7c-i). This indicates that the site of pacing is either in the inner part of the circuit itself (left, site X) or at a bystander location arising from it (right, site Y).

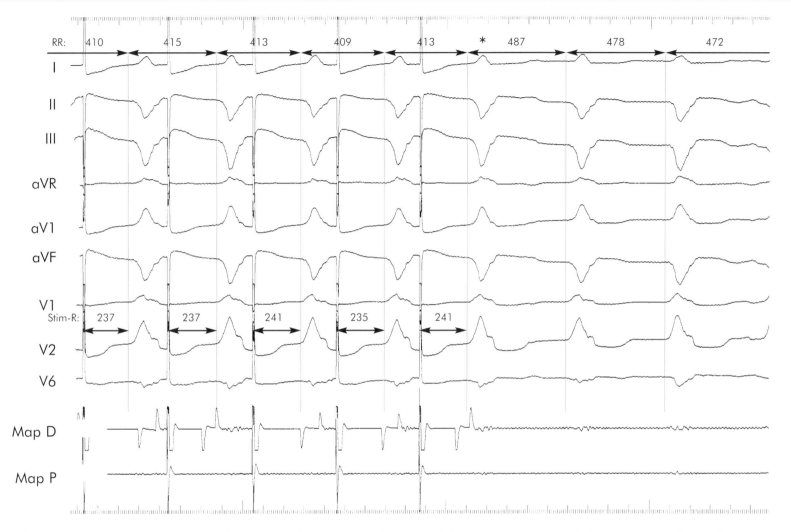

Tracing 8.7c Entrainment mapping in a patient with a large previous inferoposterior myocardial infarct and incessant VT, with a mean cycle length of 470 ms. The RBBB morphology suggests a left ventricular origin, and the axis (between −60° and −90°) suggests an inferobasal exit site. However, the site being tested is near the apex. Pacing (unipolar, hence the large stimulus artifact) is performed at this site, at a cycle length of 410 ms. RR intervals are shown at the top of the tracing. The VT is accelerated to the paced cycle length, but QRS morphology is identical to that during spontaneous tachycardia.

Note that the interval from each stimulus artifact to the resulting complex on the surface ECG (the 'stimulus time', shown lower in the tracing) is consistently well over 200 ms. During ordinary ventricular pacing, this stimulus time rarely exceeds 20–30 ms. The long stimulus time during entrainment is because the pacing site is in the zone of slow conduction (in this case, probably towards the entry site – D in Figure 8.7e), and has to travel through the zone before emerging at the exit site.

The last paced beat (*) is at the cycle length of the pace train, rather than that of the spontaneous VT. Thus, there is entrainment with concealed fusion. This indicates that the pacing site is within the zone of slow conduction, but it is not yet clear whether it is within the circuit itself or at a bystander location.

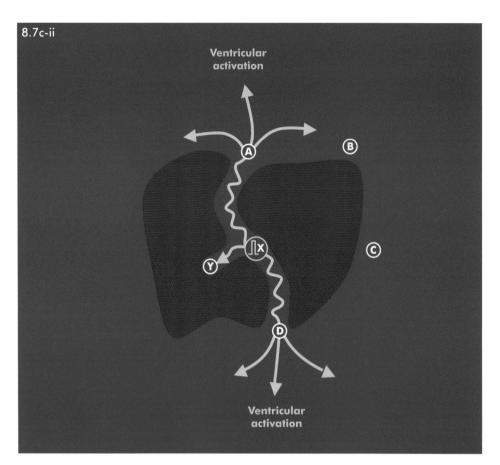

8.7c-ii

Ventricular activation

Ventricular activation

As noted above, entrainment with concealed fusion can be achieved at 'bystander' sites leading off the inner path of the circuit (Y in Figure 8.7c-i). Clearly, ablation at these locations is unlikely to be effective. Two methods can be used to determine whether an entrainment site is actually in the circuit – both depend on the extra time taken for activation to travel between the circuit itself and the bystander location.

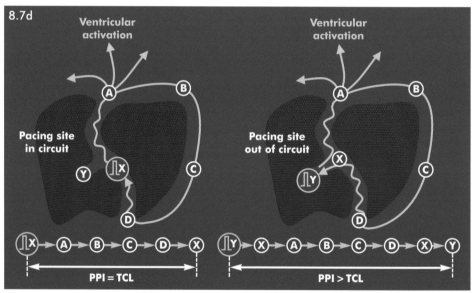

8.7d

Ventricular activation

Ventricular activation

Pacing site in circuit

Pacing site out of circuit

PPI = TCL

PPI > TCL

Note that entrainment of tachycardia with concealed fusion is possible at sites that do not give a good pace-map. When the rhythm is purely paced as opposed to entrained tachycardia, both orthodromic and antidromic propagation can occur (Figure 8.7c-ii). Thus, paced ventricular activation spreads from both the tachycardia exit site (A) and the tachycardia 'entrance' site (D). A good pace-map is usually only achieved from a location near the tachycardia exit site (A).

The *post-pacing interval* (PPI) is the time from the last entraining stimulus to the next non-stimulated depolarization, *measured at the pacing site* (Figure 8.7d). If the pacing site is in the circuit (left), the post-pacing interval is simply the time taken for the impulse to travel round the circuit, i.e. the tachycardia cycle length (TCL) (the path is X→A→B→C→D→X). If the pacing site is outside the circuit (right), the post-pacing interval is longer than the tachycardia cycle length, as it includes the time taken to travel to and from the circuit (the path is Y→X→A→B→C→D→X →Y).

8.7E COMPARISON OF STIMULUS AND ACTIVATION TIMES

At a location where entrainment with concealed fusion is seen, there is an alternative way to determine whether a catheter location is part of the circuit or at a bystander site (Figure 8.7e-i). The *activation time* (left) is the interval from local activation of the site to the subsequent QRS complex during tachycardia (i.e. Y→QRS). The *stimulus time* (right) is the interval from the paced electrogram during entrainment at the same site to the evoked QRS complex (again, Y→QRS). As shown in Figure 8.7e-i, if the site is a bystander location (Y), the stimulus time exceeds the activation time, as the paced impulse has to travel the extra distance into the circuit.

Figure 8.7e-ii illustrates that, if the site is in the circuit (X), the stimulus time equals the activation time, as the paths of paced and spontaneous activation from the site to the QRS complex are identical.

Thus, confirmation that an entraining site is in the tachycardia circuit can come from two comparisons: (i) if the post-pacing interval equals the tachycardia cycle length, or (ii) if the stimulus time (during entrainment with concealed fusion) equals the activation time (during tachycardia). In practice, neither comparison is 100% precise: a discrepancy of ~25 ms in either of these comparisons is still compatible with a location within the tachycardia circuit.

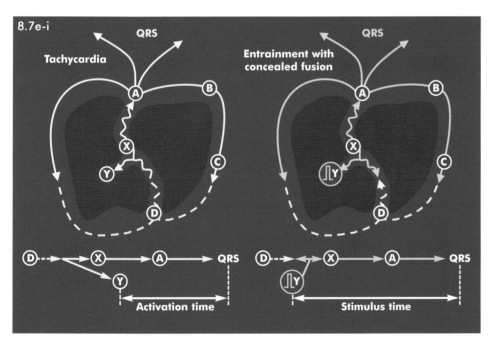

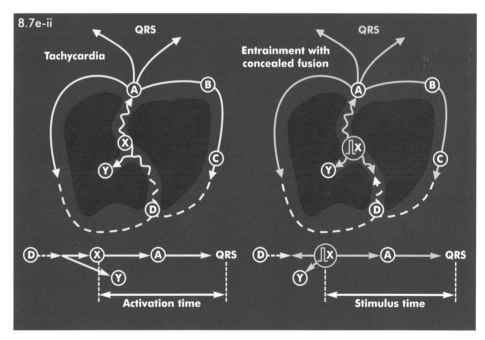

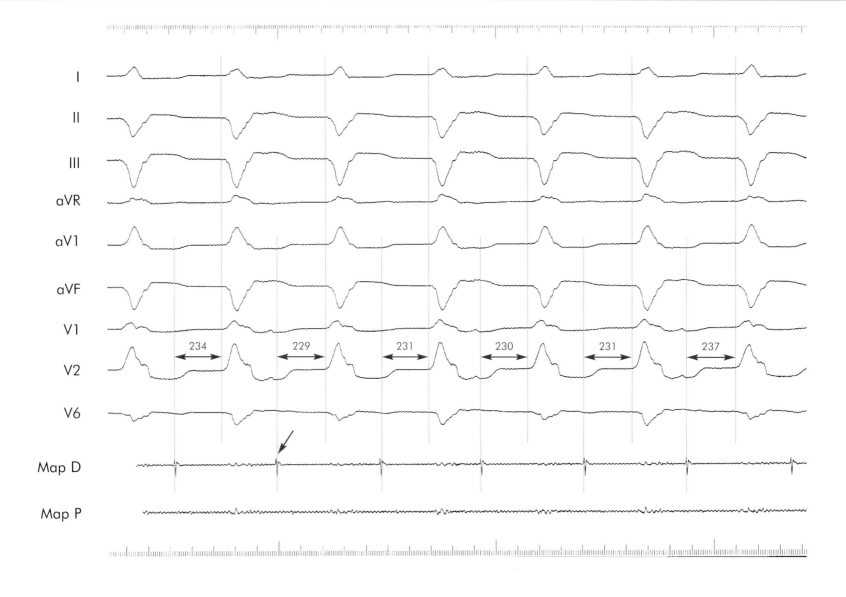

Tracing 8.7e-i At the site illustrated in Tracing 8.7c, a small, sharp diastolic potential (arrowed) is recorded from the distal bipole (Map D, highly amplified) during spontaneous VT. The activation time, measured from this potential to the QRS, is around 232 ms. This is almost identical to the 'stimulus time' noted in Tracing 8.7c. Thus, the catheter is within the common pathway of the circuit itself and not at a bystander location.

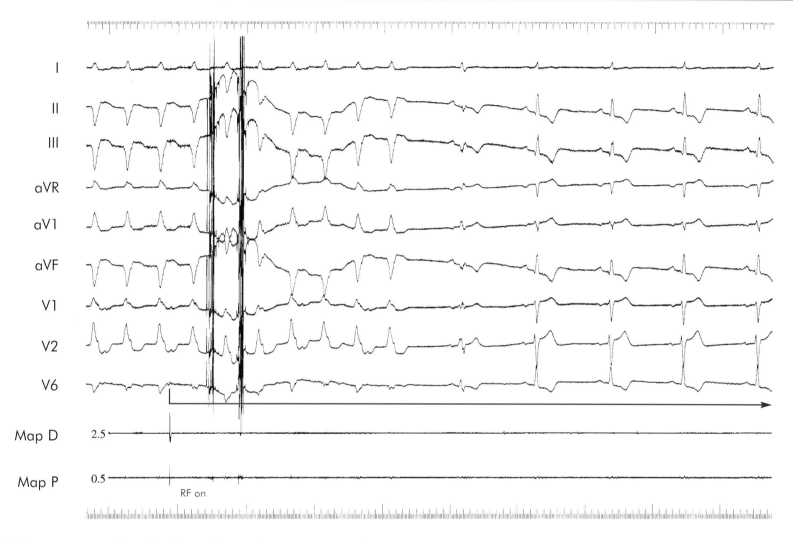

Tracing 8.7e-ii RF energy was delivered at the site illustrated in Tracings 8.7c and 8.7e-i. Tachycardia, previously incessant, terminated after 3 s. Energy delivery was continued for a full minute and further RF applications were made at adjacent locations to enlarge the area of block. VT was thereafter no longer inducible.

We have seen that different mapping tools can be used to identify functionally a location within the zone of slow conduction in the circuit (diastolic potentials and entrainment with concealed fusion), and confirm that it is not a bystander location (post-pacing interval, stimulus versus activation times). If ablation at such a location terminates tachycardia, it is customary to deliver one or two extra lesions at adjacent locations to enlarge the area of block created, then test whether the tachycardia can still be reinduced. If ablation at a site identified by entrainment mapping does not terminate tachycardia, this is probably because the tachycardia is able to bypass the lesion, as the isthmus of conduction is wide at that point. In this case, one can test another location, or attempt to draw a line of block across the functionally-defined isthmus.

The techniques described so far in this book are generally considered to constitute the conventional armamentarium of the clinical electrophysiologist. They are highly effective in diagnosis, and over the last 10 years have revolutionized the treatment of certain tachycardias – AVNRT and AVRT, and 'focal' atrial and ventricular tachycardias. However, it is fair to say that the majority of VT cases cannot yet be cured by ablation, partly because patients cannot tolerate VT for the time required for mapping using current methods, and partly because of the inability of conventional RF energy to produce controlled lesions of sufficient size. Even in the era of the implantable cardioverter defibrillator (ICD), VT remains a major clinical problem, and tools are needed that can more rapidly map and eliminate the substrate. Likewise, atypical atrial flutter and atrial fibrillation remain significant challenges to the electrophysiologist.

8.8A NEW CATHETER ABLATION SYSTEMS

Even with increased power and temperature control, insufficient lesion size can be a limitation with conventional RF ablation. The simplest way to obtain a larger lesion is by increasing the catheter tip length. This increases the degree to which circulating blood cools the tip, and enables a higher current to be delivered to the tissue for the same catheter/tissue interface temperature. An 8-mm tip catheter can create a lesion of up to four times the volume of a 4-mm tip catheter (Figure 8.8a-i). This is usually sufficient to achieve, for example, full-thickness lesions across pectinate muscle in the subeustachian isthmus for flutter ablation, where a 4-mm tip may fail. An even greater degree of cooling, and hence a larger lesion size, may be achieved using a saline-irrigated catheter tip (Figure 8.8a-ii).

For the purpose of creating linear atrial lesions, catheters with multiple ablation electrodes over a length of several centimeters have been developed (Figure 8.8a-iii) – it appears likely that each segment will need separate temperature control to achieve continuous transmural lesions while avoiding charring.

Examples of new catheter types are shown in Figure 8.8a. (i) conventional 4-mm tip RF catheter and 8-mm tip RF catheter side-by-side in the right atrium (Conductr™ 4mm and Conductr™ 8mm), (ii) irrigated tip RF catheter (Sprinklr™), (iii) linear ablation RF catheter with six coil electrodes (Amazr™ Sidewindr). Courtesy of Medtronic, Inc (Cardiorhythm Division).

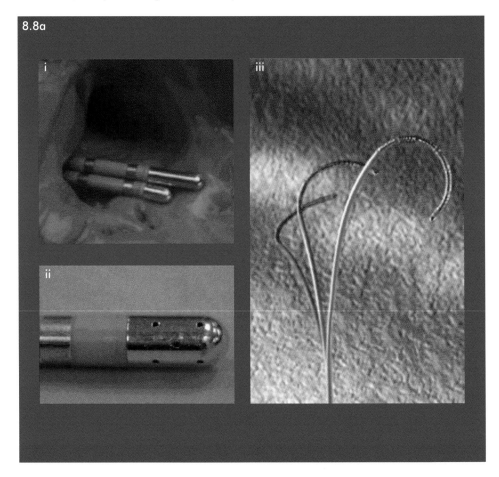

8.8a

Other energy sources that are being investigated include laser, microwave, cryoablation and ultrasound.

Unlike most *laser* sources, the neodymium-yttrium-argon (Nd-YAG) laser penetrates tissue and can cause volume heating if applied over several seconds. The system requires a costly energy source and requires good optical contact with tissue (excluding blood), but holds promise.

Microwave sources have been shown to produce lesions far greater in volume than conventional RF, and do not require tissue contact. The chief limitations of microwave energy are obtaining control of the direction of the radiated energy (perpendicular to the catheter tip, rather than axial), and transmission power loss that causes heating of the shaft.

Cryoablation has been used since the earliest days of electrophysiologic surgery. The lesion produced is discrete, less disruption of tissue architecture and scarring are produced than with RF, and there is apparently no risk of endocardial charring and clot formation. Another substantial advantage of cryoablation is that moderate cooling (0°C to –20°C) seems to produce effects in the tissue that are largely reversible, and thus 'ice-mapping' can be performed to identify a target location, where an irreversible lesion is formed at temperatures below –40°C. Cryoablation has only hitherto been possible in the operating room, as it requires a large hand-held probe for expansion of gas. However, steerable catheters have been developed for percutaneous use, employing either gaseous or liquid refrigerants.

Figure 8.8a-iv. Left: cryoablation catheter with 4-mm tip. Right: the same catheter with an iceball formed at the tip. This appearance is slightly misleading: *in vivo*, circulating blood prevents iceball formation within the cardiac chambers, and only the myocardium itself is frozen. Illustration courtesy of Cryocath, Inc.

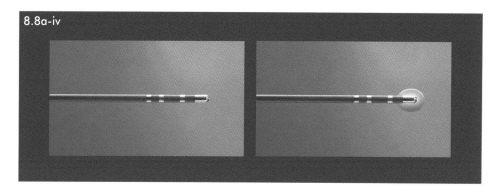

8.8a-iv

Finally, *ultrasound* may offer similar advantages to cryoablation, obtaining tissue necrosis without the need for high temperatures and the risks of char and clot formation. Depending on the transducer used, energy can be directed forward from the tip of the catheter, or in a perpendicular direction. A fluid-filled balloon catheter has been developed to plug the orifice of a pulmonary vein while ultrasound energy is directed equatorially. This is intended to create a ring lesion, isolating the vein and any ectopy arising therein from the left atrium.

Current standard mapping systems are more than adequate for the electrophysiological procedures described in this book. However, because of certain shortcomings, some arrhythmias remain difficult to treat by catheter ablation. Firstly, conventional methods record from only a few locations in the heart – usually a few fixed references and a single mapping catheter. To build up a picture of an arrhythmia, this catheter must explore the heart while local activation is compared with a reference at each location. This requires the arrhythmia to be both sustained and stable, which is not always the case. Moreover, only a minority of patients with scar-related VT can tolerate the arrhythmia for the length of time required for mapping. Single ectopic beats and short runs of focal ectopy can be very difficult to localize, especially when they only occur sporadically. Secondly, conventional systems are limited in their ability to build up an 'electro-anatomical map', identifying activation times and mapping catheter locations with real positions in space, and remembering where lesions have been created. Finally, conventional mapping is time-consuming and can involve long fluoroscopy times, putting both patient and operator at some risk from radiation exposure.

Newer mapping systems take advantage of the prodigious recent advances in hardware capacity and software design to rapidly build up representations of cardiac chambers, and to generate maps of electrical activation, electrogram voltage and catheter locations (and thus ablation lesion locations) in three dimensions. More than one approach has been taken.

The 'basket' catheter is a percutaneous version of the balloon and sock arrays that have been used for endocardial and epicardial surgical mapping of arrhythmias for several years (Figure 8.8b-i, courtesy of Boston Scientific/EP Technologies). A large number of electrodes are arranged on a number of splines that expand into a basket-like array when deployed from a sheath. (In this figure, a basket catheter with 64 electrodes arranged on 8 splines [A–H] has been deployed in the right atrium in a patient undergoing isthmus ablation for atrial flutter.)

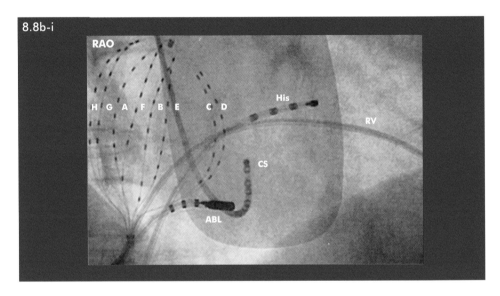

8.8b-i

Endocardial contact electrograms from each electrode are processed by the computer station and displayed either in a conventional manner or as isochronal maps. By using a large number of electrodes, global activation of the chamber can be mapped. The activation of each beat is recorded over the whole array. Thus, an ectopic focus or the exit site of a VT circuit can in theory be identified from a single beat, eliminating the need for stable, sustained tachycardia. Furthermore, by emitting an identification signal, the location of the mapping catheter in relation to the basket array can be determined. This can be used to build up an anatomically correct image of the endocardial surface, to guide the mapping catheter to a region of interest, and to display locations of interest (e.g. ablation sites). A shortcoming of the basket catheter concept is that the complex morphology of the cardiac chambers may make it difficult to achieve good tissue contact with all the electrodes.

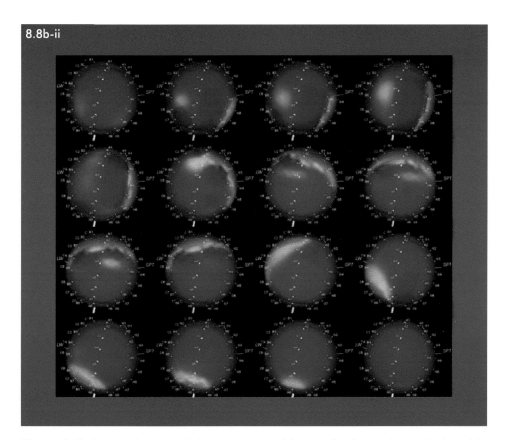

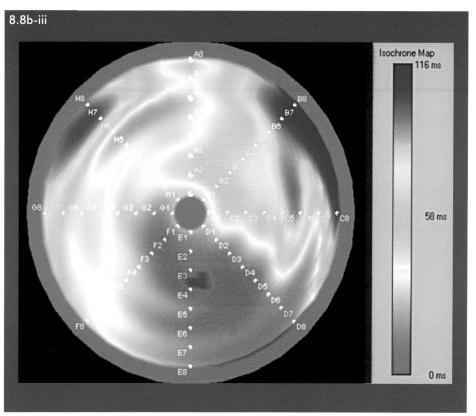

Figure 8.8b-ii is an isopotential map obtained from a basket catheter deployed in the right atrium during atrial flutter. Activation is seen to emerge from the subeustachian isthmus in the first frames, ascend the interatrial septum (SPT) to the roof in frames 4–8, and descend the lateral wall (LW) in frames 9–14 before re-entering the isthmus. (Courtesy of Cathdata, Inc.)

Figure 8.8b-iii is an isochronal activation map obtained from a basket catheter in the right atrium. Activation is seen to emanate from a focus located in the vicinity of poles E3 and E4. (Courtesy of Cathdata, Inc.)

Non-fluoroscopic mapping allows the location of a mapping catheter to be computed in three dimensions without X-rays, using an electromagnetic field generated by sources external to the patient and detected by the catheter itself. As the catheter is moved around a cardiac chamber, its location is stored by a computer simultaneously with the local electrogram, and a map of endocardial activation within that chamber can gradually be built up, point-by-point. This requires that the rhythm being mapped remains stable over a few minutes at least.

Figure 8.8b-iv shows a sequence of illustrations of atypical flutter related to a previous atriotomy scar. The atrium is viewed from behind, the green and grey rings indicate the origins of the superior and inferior venae cavae, and the yellow bar indicates the proximal coronary sinus. The red areas indicate the wavefront of depolarization, which propagates in a 'figure of eight' fashion between and around two inexcitable islands of tissue (large and small grey areas). Courtesy of Biosense Webster CARTO and Drs Hebe and Kuck.

One form of *non-contact mapping* uses a multi-electrode array mounted on a balloon catheter situated in the cavity of the heart chamber. Instead of recording electrograms by direct contact, the array detects the endocavitary electrical field generated by cardiac activation and mathematically reconstructs the endocardial potentials responsible for generating that field. Like the basket, this offers the ability to map global endocardial activation of a cardiac chamber from a single beat, but it is not dependent on tissue contact. There are certain limitations to this concept: the system is contingent on the ability to keep the balloon catheter stable in the chamber being mapped, and the reconstructed electrograms are unreliable when the distance from balloon to endocardium exceeds ~3 cm.

Figure 8.8b-v shows an intracavitary balloon catheter used for non-contact mapping. The balloon is inflated, deploying the multi-electrode array formed from a mesh of wires on its surface. Courtesy of ESI.

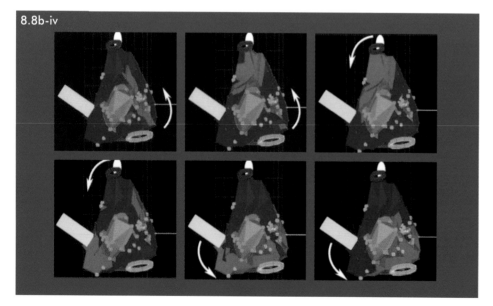

8.8b-iv

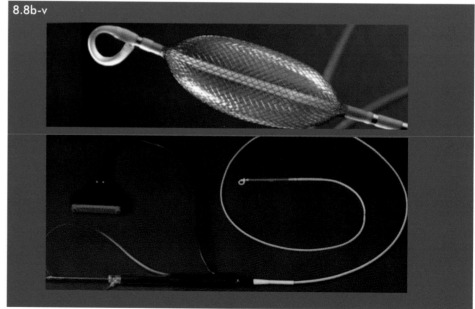

8.8b-v

Figure 8.8b-vi shows ventricular tachycardia recorded from the left ventricular cavity using a non-contact multi-electrode array. The ventricle has been opened to show the entire endocardial surface. Frame 1 shows the emergence of activation from the diastolic pathway at the exit site. Frames 2–4 show rapid systolic activation of the ventricle, followed by entry into the diastolic pathway (arrowed, Frame 4). Frames 5–8 show slow progress of activation along the diastolic pathway to the exit site. (Reproduced with permission from Schilling RJ et al. Circulation 1999;99:2543–2552.)

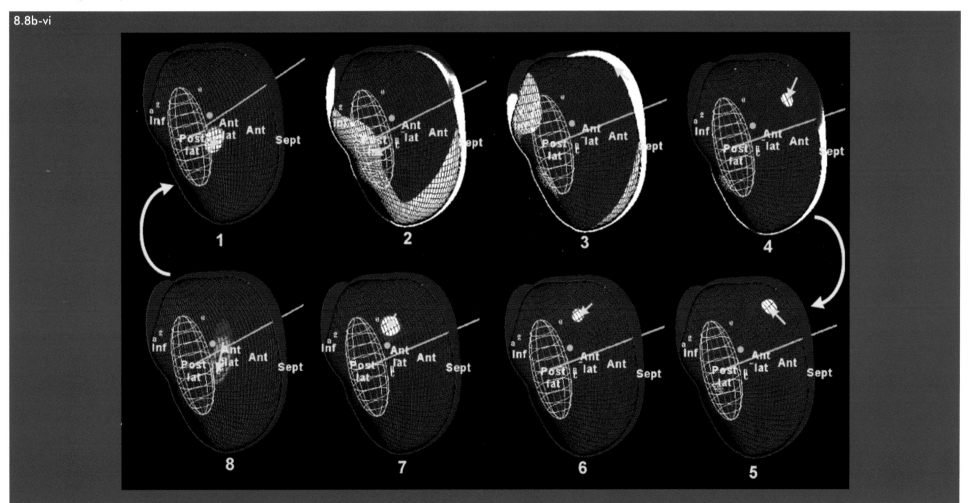

8.8b-vi

FURTHER READING

1. Haines DE. The biophysics and pathophysiology of lesion formation during radiofrequency catheter ablation. In: Zipes DP, Jalife J. Cardiac Electrophysiology: From Cell to Bedside. Philadelphia: WB Saunders, 1999:983–93.

2. Touboul P. Atrioventricular nodal ablation and pacemaker implantation in patients with atrial fibrillation. Am J Cardiol 1999;83(5B):241D–245D.

3. Narasimhan C, Blanck Z, Akhtar M. Atrioventricular nodal modification and atrioventricular junctional ablation for control of ventricular rate in atrial fibrillation. J Cardiovasc Electrophysiol 1998;9(8 Suppl.):S146–50.

4. Haissaguerre M, Jais P, Shah DC et al. Analysis of electrophysiological activity in Koch's triangle relevant to ablation of the slow AV nodal pathway. Pacing Clin Electrophysiol 1997;20(10 Pt 1):2470–81.

5. Kottkamp H, Hindricks G, Borggrefe M et al. Radiofrequency catheter ablation of the anterosuperior and posteroinferior atrial approaches to the AV node for treatment of AV nodal reentrant tachycardia: techniques for selective ablation of 'fast' and 'slow' AV node pathways. J Cardiovasc Electrophysiol 1997;8(4):451–68.

6. Calkins H, Yong P, Miller JM et al. Catheter ablation of accessory pathways, atrioventricular nodal reentrant tachycardia, and the atrioventricular junction: final results of a prospective, multicenter clinical trial. The Atakr Multicenter Investigators Group. Circulation 1999;99(2):262–70.

7. Jackman WM, Wang XZ, Friday KJ et al. Catheter ablation of accessory atrioventricular pathways (Wolff-Parkinson-White syndrome) by radiofrequency current. N Engl J Med 1991;324(23):1605–11.

8. Calkins H, Sousa J, el-Atassi R et al. Diagnosis and cure of the Wolff-Parkinson-White syndrome or paroxysmal supraventricular tachycardias during a single electrophysiologic test. N Engl J Med 1991;324(23):1612–8.

9. Shah DC, Haissaguerre M, Jais P et al. Atrial flutter: contemporary electrophysiology and catheter ablation. Pacing Clin Electrophysiol 1999;22(2):344–59.

10. Stevenson WG. Ventricular tachycardia after myocardial infarction: from arrhythmia surgery to catheter ablation. J Cardiovasc Electrophysiol 1995;6(10 Pt 2):942–50.

11. Lustgarten DL, Keane D, Ruskin J. Cryothermal ablation: mechanism of tissue injury and current experience in the treatment of tachyarrhythmias. Prog Cardiovasc Dis 1999;41(6):481–98.

12. Schmitt C, Zrenner B, Schneider M et al. Clinical experience with a novel multielectrode basket catheter in right atrial tachycardias. Circulation 1999;99(18):2414–22.

13. Schilling RJ, Peters NS, Davies DW. Feasibility of a noncontact catheter for endocardial mapping of human ventricular tachycardia. Circulation 1999;99(19):2543–52.

14. Varanasi S, Dhala A, Blanck Z et al. Electroanatomic mapping for radiofrequency ablation of cardiac arrhythmias. J Cardiovasc Electrophysiol 1999;10(4):538–44.

The text of this book provides the 'mechanics' of electrophysiology (EP) assessment and the fundamental concepts required to carry out and interpret the study. The following comments may assist in establishing a philosophical framework for a successful study. It goes without saying that the successful electrophysiologist has a good knowledge base, sound technical skills and good instincts for arrhythmia diagnosis. Beyond this, it is important to have a systematic approach to the study and interpretation of the observations. A careful review of all the patient's records should result in a reasonable preliminary differential diagnosis. The EP study should be standardized for the given problem with an orderly plan of programmed stimulation [1,2]. It is important to have an open mind but one generally sees what one is looking for and is prepared for opportunities to make the difficult diagnosis by an astute observation or a well-timed intervention.

Focused concentration is the order of the day. An effort to explain all observations as they unfold helps this process even if the importance of the detail seems irrelevant at the time. This trains the mind for clarity and attention to detail. It is especially productive to pay attention to transitions such as the onset or termination of a tachycardia or points of irregularity where the monotony of the arrhythmia is disturbed by change in cycle length or QRS morphology.

Proceed from the general to the specific. Analyze the surface ECG recordings before looking at the intracardiacs. As Mark E Josephson teaches, look on the 'outside of the heart' first. Clinical electrophysiology is essentially electrocardiography but more powerful because of additional intracardiac recordings and the ability to perturb the system with stimulation or pharmacological interventions. List the differential diagnosis for the observation in question and proceed to compile the evidence to eliminate the incorrect ones [3]. This is basically an exercise in hypothesis testing [4]. Consider additional pacing, autonomic or pharmacological maneuvers that will support or clarify the favored hypothesis.

Approach to the unknown EP tracing

• General overview

• Analyze the surface ECG

• Analyze the intracardiac records

• What is the A to V relationship?

• What is the atrial activation sequence?

• What is the ventricular activation sequence as determined from available sites?

• Is the His deflection visible, and what is its relation to A and V? What are the apparent HV and VA intervals?

• Formulate a hypothesis and see if it fits all the observations

Figure 9a (annotated in Figure 9b) was recorded from a young woman undergoing EP study for paroxysmal atrial fibrillation and provides an illustration of these principles. The arrhythmia occurred spontaneously. Although the diagnosis may be obvious at a glance to some, it is a useful to go through the exercise. Even the most experienced electrophysiologists will make mental errors when they abbreviate the thought process and stab at the diagnosis. The surface leads are examined first followed by the intracardiac recordings.

The tracing is a 'wide QRS tachycardia' and the initial broad differential diagnosis is as follows:

1. Ventricular tachycardia (see Section 7)

2. Supraventricular tachycardia with aberrant conduction (see Section 6.5)

3. Pre-excited tachycardia (anterograde conduction over an accessory pathway) (see Section 6.8)

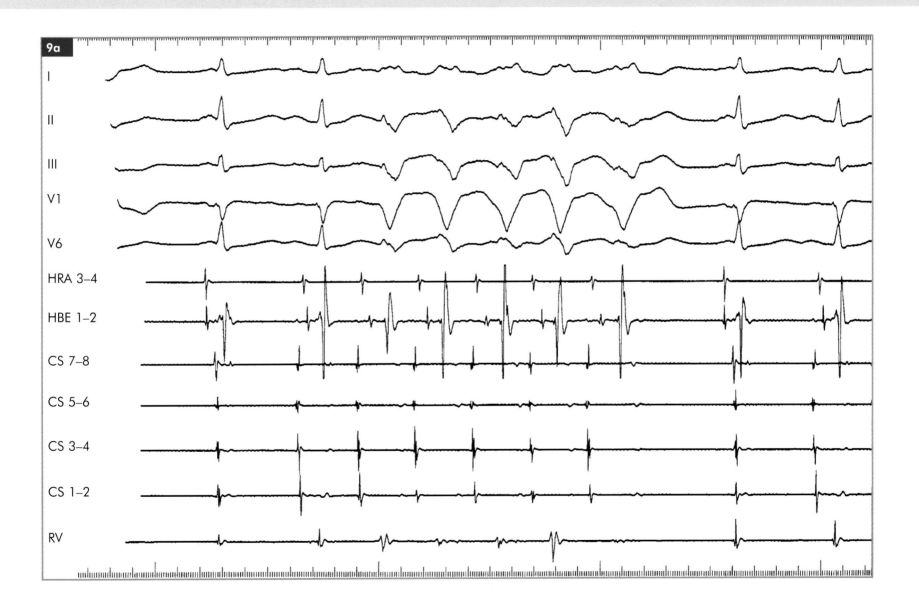

Examine the annotated version of the tracing (Tracing 9b). The surface ECG leads show a fairly 'typical' left bundle branch block pattern suggestive of aberrant conduction. The first premature cycle (first cycle of the run, asterisked) has supraventricular morphology and is preceded by a P-wave, again suggesting that the run is supraventricular. The intracardiac recordings indicate a one-to-one A–V relationship with atrial activity accompanying ventricular activity. Furthermore, a His deflection precedes each QRS and the HV interval is of normal duration (50 ms). For all practical purposes, this rules out ventricular tachycardia.

The diagnosis is narrowed to supraventricular tachycardia. The differential diagnosis is further refined to:

1. Sinus tachycardia (see Section 3.1)

2. Atrial tachycardia (see Section 3.2)

3. Junctional reentrant tachycardia (AV nodal reentry, Section 4.2 or AV reentry Section 5.4)

The atrial activation sequence is then examined. Atrial activation is generally classified as: (i) sinus (normal), with the high right atrium near sinus node activated first; or (ii) ectopic (abnormal), which is anything other than sinus. When atrial activation is thought to be retrograde proceeding from the ventricles or AV junction, it is classified as 'concentric' (AV node region at HB catheter first) or 'eccentric' with earliest atrial activation at an AV ring site other than the AV node region.

In Figure 9b, initial inspection of the surface ECG shows the abnormal P-wave of the first cycle of tachycardia (arrowed). The P-wave is upright in leads 2 and 3, indicating a 'high-to-low' activation pattern. This in itself rules out a junctional reentrant tachycardia because it is not compatible with retrograde conduction from the AV node or the ventricles. Examining the intracardiac recordings, earliest atrial activation (A*) occurs at the left paraseptal region in the coronary sinus (CS 5–6). This rules out sinus tachycardia, which would also have a 'high-to-low' pattern but would begin in the high right atrium.

If one looks more closely at the atrial activation sequence on the intracardiac recordings, one notes that all the CS atrial electrograms are activated nearly simultaneously even though CS 5–6 is earliest. It is noted that each of the CS electrodes are 10 mm apart and can only be activated simultaneously from a distant site relatively equidistant to each of the recording electrodes. The right atrial electrogram is relatively late, strongly suggesting that the ectopic focus is in the left atrium and indeed in the high left atrium. In this example, it was subsequently ablated in the right upper pulmonary vein.

In this process, we have listed the diagnostic possibilities, beginning with a broad differential diagnosis and expanding to more specific diagnoses. In the end, we eliminated all the possibilities except the correct one, which was a left atrial tachycardia (so called 'ectopic' atrial tachycardia). We may then ask what we would have done if recordings from the 'routine' study did not yield the diagnosis.

Reproducible induction or presence of tachycardia allows one to manipulate it with autonomic, pharmacological or stimulation maneuvers. Adenosine is very useful and usually allows one to distinguish a tachycardia that doesn't require the AV node (i.e. atrial tachycardia) from a junctional reentrant tachycardia. Atrial tachycardias may terminate with adenosine but will frequently exhibit AV block prior to termination. Ventricular extrastimuli or burst ventricular pacing during tachycardia are very useful in establishing the role of the ventricles in the tachycardia mechanism. The mechanism of tachycardia can be invariably established with a systematic approach.

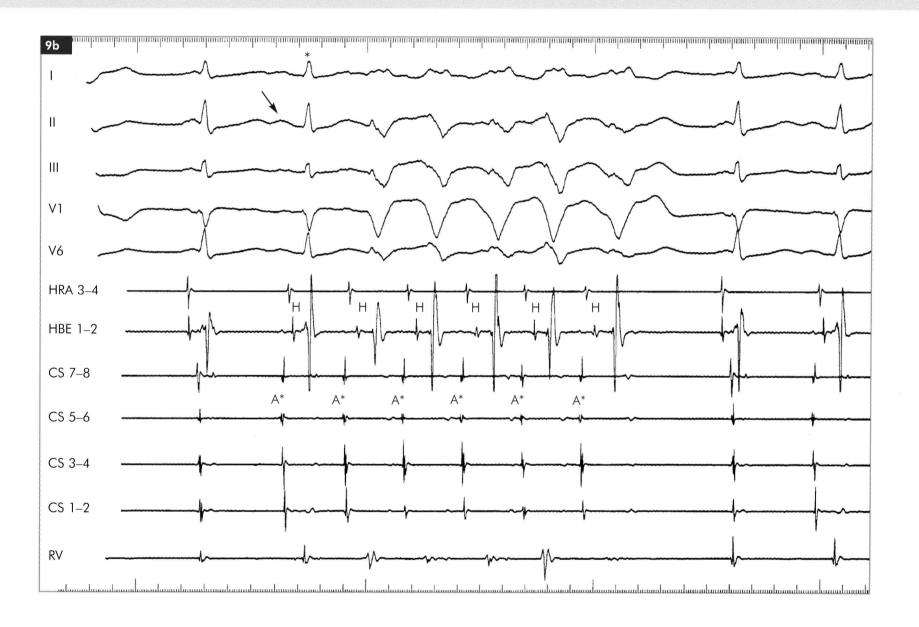

The following is a list of differential diagnoses that should be considered when examining an unknown EP tracing of tachycardia. These are shown diagrammatically in Figure 9c.

DIFFERENTIAL DIAGNOSIS OF WIDE QRS TACHYCARDIA

1. Ventricular tachycardia (see Section 7)
2. Supraventricular tachycardia (SVT) with aberrancy (see Section 6.5)
3. Pre-excited tachycardia (see Section 6.8)

DIFFERENTIAL DIAGNOSIS OF NARROW QRS TACHYCARDIA

1. Atrial tachycardia (see Section 3.2)
2. AV nodal reentry (see Section 4.2)
3. AV reentry (see Section 5.4)
4. Junctional tachycardia (see Section 6.4E)
5. Ventricular tachycardia (very rare forms: fascicular tachycardia [idiopathic left ventricle (LV) ventricular tachycardia (VT)], 'septal' VT which can mimic SVT) (see Section 7.4)

CONCENTRIC ATRIAL ACTIVATION SEQUENCE DURING TACHYCARDIA

Narrow QRS
1. Atrial tachycardia (originating near the AV node) (see Section 3.2)
2. AV nodal reentry (see Section 4.2)
3. AV reentry (pathway near the AV node) (see Section 5.4)
4. Junctional tachycardia (see Section 6.4E)

Wide QRS
1. SVT (as for narrow QRS) with aberrancy (see Sections 3–6)
2. Pre-excited tachycardia (antidromic tachycardia) (see Section 6.8)
3. VT with VA conduction (see Section 7)

ECCENTRIC ATRIAL ACTIVATION SEQUENCE DURING TACHYCARDIA

Narrow QRS complex
1. Atrial tachycardia (see Section 3.2)
2. AV reentry (see Section 5.4)

Wide QRS complex
1. SVT (as for narrow QRS) with aberrancy (see Section 6.5)
2. Pre-excited tachycardia (see Section 6.8)
3. VT (see Section 7)

ABSENT H OR 'SHORT' HV INTERVAL DURING TACHYCARDIA

1. VT (see Section 7)
2. Pre-excited tachycardia (see Section 6.8)
3. Inappropriate His recording site

PRE-EXCITED TACHYCARDIA: CONCENTRIC ATRIAL ACTIVATION

AP part of tachycardia circuit
1. Antidromic reentry (including atriofascicular type) (see Section 6.8C)
2. Pathway-to-pathway reentry (see Section 6.8E)
3. Nodoventricular or nodofascicular reentry (see Section 5.8A)

AP not part of tachycardia circuit ('bystander' conduction)
1. Atrial tachycardia (see Section 6.8B)
2. AV nodal reentry (see Section 6.8B)

PRE-EXCITED TACHYCARDIA: ECCENTRIC ATRIAL ACTIVATION

AP part of tachycardia circuit
  Pathway-to-pathway reentry (see Section 6.8E)
AP not part of tachycardia circuit
  Atrial tachycardia (see Section 6.8B)

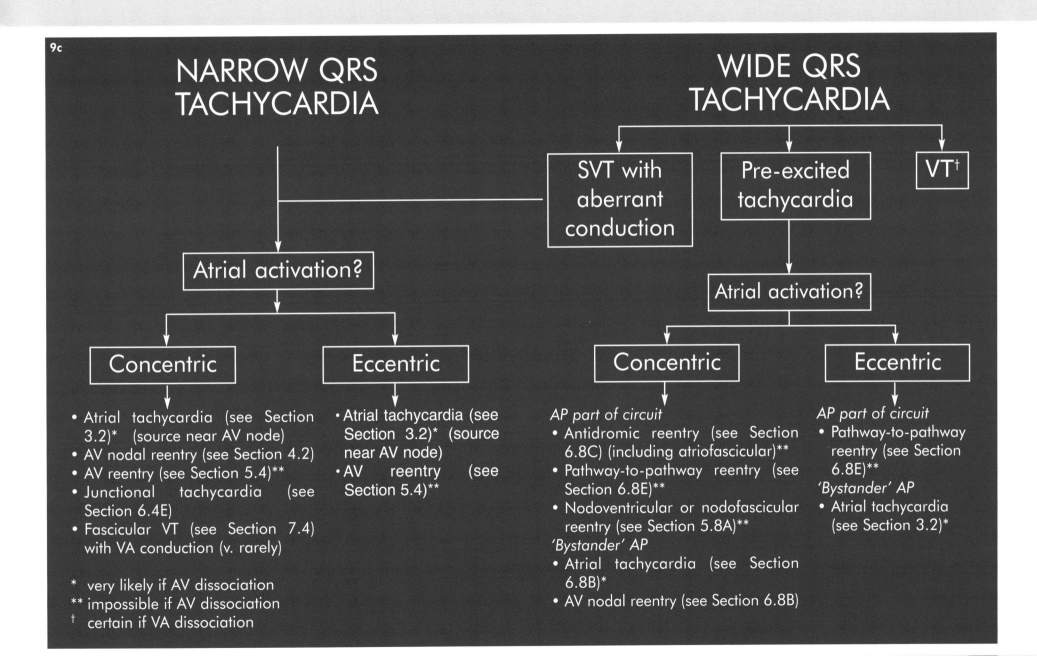

NARROW QRS TACHYCARDIA

WIDE QRS TACHYCARDIA

SVT with aberrant conduction

Pre-excited tachycardia

VT†

Atrial activation?

Atrial activation?

Concentric

Eccentric

Concentric

Eccentric

- Atrial tachycardia (see Section 3.2)* (source near AV node)
- AV nodal reentry (see Section 4.2)
- AV reentry (see Section 5.4)**
- Junctional tachycardia (see Section 6.4E)
- Fascicular VT (see Section 7.4) with VA conduction (v. rarely)

- Atrial tachycardia (see Section 3.2)* (source near AV node)
- AV reentry (see Section 5.4)**

AP part of circuit
- Antidromic reentry (see Section 6.8C) (including atriofascicular)**
- Pathway-to-pathway reentry (see Section 6.8E)**
- Nodoventricular or nodofascicular reentry (see Section 5.8A)**

'Bystander' AP
- Atrial tachycardia (see Section 6.8B)*
- AV nodal reentry (see Section 6.8B)

AP part of circuit
- Pathway-to-pathway reentry (see Section 6.8E)**

'Bystander' AP
- Atrial tachycardia (see Section 3.2)*

* very likely if AV dissociation
** impossible if AV dissociation
† certain if VA dissociation

9c

237

The values given below are derived from a survey of the literature, and should in most cases be viewed as an indication of expected values rather than absolute cut-offs. Reference ranges used by other EP laboratories may differ slightly from these values. Furthermore, many of these measures are extremely sensitive to functional factors, e.g. cycle length, autonomic tone and presence of anti-arrhythmic and anesthetic drugs.

CONDUCTION INTERVALS

PA	25–55 ms
AH	55–125 ms
HBE duration	<30 ms
HV	35–55 ms
QRS	≤100 ms
QTc	Men: ≤450 ms (borderline if 430–450 ms)
	Women: ≤470 ms (borderline if 450–470 ms)

SINUS NODE FUNCTION

Maximum SNRT	≤1.5 s
CSNRT	<550 ms
Maximum TRT	≤5 s
SACT	50–115 ms

REFRACTORY PERIODS

Atrial ERP	180–330 ms
AV Nodal ERP	250–400 ms (antegrade conduction)
AV Nodal FRP	330–550 ms
Ventricular ERP	180–290 ms

1. Josephson ME. Clinical Cardiac Electrophysiology: Techniques and Interpretations. Philadelphia/London: Lea and Febiger, 1993.

2. Prystowsky EN, Klein GJ. In J Dereck, editor. Cardiac Arrhythmia: An Integrated Approach for the Clinician. New York: McGraw-Hill, 1994.

3. Klein GJ, Prystowsky EN. Clinical Electrophysiology Review. New York: McGraw Hill, 1997.

4. Teo WS, Yee R, Klein GJ et al. Hypothesis testing as an approach to the analysis of complex tachycardias – An illustrative case of a preexcitation variant. PACE 1991;14(10):1503–13.

W

Wenckebach cycle length (WCL) 28, 48–49, 51–52, 59

Wolff-Parkinson-White syndrome, mortality risk 146

Z

zone of reset, SACT 22–23

zone of slow conduction, catheter activation mapping 217